COLOR ATLAS OF C.S.F. CYTOPATHOLOGY

COLOR ATLAS OF C.S.F. CYTOPATHOLOGY

W.A. den Hartog Jager
Professor of Neurology (emeritus)
Wilhelmina Gasthuis, Department of Experimental Neurology,
Municipal University of Amsterdam, The Netherlands

With a chapter on immunofluorescence of C.S.F. cells
by A.C.B. Peters[1] and J. Versteeg[2]

[1] Department of Neurology and [2] Laboratory of Medical
Microbiology, University Hospital of Leiden, The Netherlands

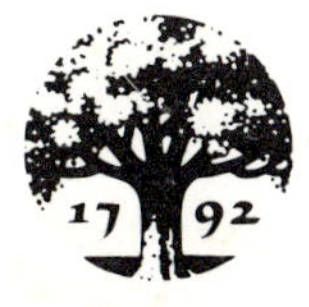

J.B. LIPPINCOTT COMPANY
PHILADELPHIA • TORONTO

ISBN Elsevier/North-Holland 0-444-80210-×
ISBN Lippincott: 0-397-58265-×

Published by:
Elsevier/North-Holland Biomedical Press
335 Jan van Galenstraat, P.O. Box 211
Amsterdam, The Netherlands

Sole distributors for the USA and Canada:
J.B. Lippincott Company
E. Washington Sq.
Philadelphia, PA 19105
U.S.A.

Library of Congress Cataloging in Publication Data

```
Hartog Jager, W    A    den.
   Color atlas of C.S.F. cytopathology.

   Bibliography:  p.
   1.  Cerebrospinal fluid--Examination--Atlases.
2.  Diagnosis, Cytologic--Atlases.  3.  Pathology,
Cellular--Atlases.  I.  Peters, A.C.B.  II.  Versteeg,
Jan, lector.  III.  Title.  [DNLM: 1.  Cerebrospinal
fluid--Cytology--Atlases.  2.  Central nervous system
diseases--Pathology--Atlases.  3.  Central nervous
system diseases--Cerebrospinal fluid--Atlases.
QY17 H334c]
RB55.H34     616.07'582     80-11491
ISBN 0-444-80210-X (Elsevier/North-Holland Biomedial
Press)
ISBN 0-397-58265-X (Lippincott)
```

PRINTED IN THE NETHERLANDS

Dedicated to my wife, Milly.

Contents

Index of color photographs

Index of black and white photographs

Preface

This color atlas of C.S.F. (cerebrospinal fluid) cytopathology is written to aid the uninitiated in this branch of neurology. The author has made use of his own experience, and of the work of other scientists in the field, as mentioned in the text and references.

Neurology has always been a science in which, in the words of Szent-Gyorgi, 'more brains and less hardware' have been significant. Radiology and its latest offspring - the computer-assisted tomography - have become so important that the younger generation of neurologists is inclined to underestimate the value of bedside diagnosis and examination of the spinal fluid. There are, however, many immunological and morphological findings in C.S.F., which can lead directly to the diagnosis, thereby saving the patient from superfluous, unpleasant and expensive examinations.

The color atlas has been written with this in mind, and if it succeeds, the work will not have been in vain.

Acknowledgements

My venerated teacher, Prof. A. Biemond, stimulated my interest in the cytopathology of the C.S.F.

In 1962, Dr. Bots from Leiden instructed me in the Sayk technique for which I am very grateful.

The material came from the Neurological Department, (heads: formerly, Professor A. Biemond and, subsequently, myself), and the Neurosurgical Department (heads: formerly, Professor W. Noordenbos and, now, Professor A.J.M. van der Werf), Municipal University, Amsterdam.

The C.S.F. cell preparations were made with unflagging enthusiasm by the head technicians Miss E. Hische and Miss A. Tutuarima.

For many instructive evenings in general cytopathology, I am grateful to Dr. Lopez Cardozo, whose knowledge in this field is, in my opinion, unsurpassed in the Netherlands. Dr. Peters and Dr. Versteeg have extended the book with their chapter on immunofluorescence. Dr. Hoogendijk kindly supplied some photographs of bacterial meningitis.

The help of Miss Maathuis with preparation of the microphotographs was of the greatest value.

The secretarial work was performed by Miss Goossens with diligence and enthusiasm.

There are many unmentioned colleagues who, in the course of 17 years, have helped by asking questions, or at least saying a kind word.

Abbreviations

L.C.S.F. = lumbar cerebrospinal fluid
S.C.S.F. = suboccipital cerebrospinal fluid
V.C.S.F. = ventricular cerebrospinal fluid
F.I.T.C. = fluorescein isothiocyanate

Color photographs

Carl Zeiss photomicroscope with semi-automatic exposure apparatus. Planapo objectives.

Film: Agfachrome 50 L. Professional 135-36 (Agfa).

Photographic apparatus - Zeiss Ikon.

Magnification

Magnification color transparencies - color photograph - 2.7 ×.

Staining

Jenner-Giemsa, unless otherwise stated.

Chapter 1

Introduction

Since the first paper on C.S.F. cytopathology by Widal, Ravaut and Siccard in 1901, many articles on this subject have appeared. Larger works have been published by Sayk (1960), Dufresne (1973), Kölmel (1976) and Oehmichen (1976). However, many of the original papers in journals are repetitions, and often their illustrations in black and white are not particularly instructive, especially about tumor cells.

Two principal questions dominate the field of C.S.F. cytology. The first is how to develop the best technique to make as many C.S.F. cells as possible available for examination, whilst keeping them in the best possible state of preservation in order to retain even the finest cellular details. The second is how simple staining techniques may be used to provide most of the answers to questions posed by clinicians.

As to the first question the following techniques are employed by the majority of workers:

a) the sedimentation method (after Sayk);
b) Millipore or Nucleopore filtration methods (membrane filter techniques);
c) the centrifugal method.

The finer details of cells are best preserved by the sedimentation method, but cell loss is greatest with this technique.

Special staining methods have been used in attempts to solve the second problem; for example Sudan III and Sudan black B for fat, Best's carmine for glycogen, PAS, Alcian blue or Alcian green for mucopolysaccharides, enzymatic reactions, e.g. acid and alkaline phosphatase, Dopa, and Schmorl staining for melanin, and the Berlin blue reaction for iron.

Specific results can only be obtained from Schmorl and Dopa reactions for melanin, acid phosphatase in cases of prostatic carcinoma and PAS or Alcian blue staining of mucus in cases of adenocarcinoma.

Methods for electron microscopic study of C.S.F. cells are given by Duffy et al. (1969) and Herndon et al. (1974).

Herndon et al. also described mumps viral nucleocapsoid-like material in ependymal cells, choroid plexus cells and lymphocytes in the spinal fluid. They found herpes-like particles in mononuclear cells in the C.S.F. in a case of herpes zoster.

Techniques must be developed so that electron microscope findings may be presented to the clinician within 24 hours or less. This has already been done in instances of cytomegalovirus infection of cells in the urine (Lee et al. 1978).

Cell cultures give no information of direct and practical diagnostic significance although they may be of great importance in pure research. The technique of specific immunofluorescent antigens in different types of viral meningitis promises much for the near future. In bacterial meningitis the older established staining methods for bacteria are of lasting value.

In this atlas only those techniques are discussed which have been used by the author and have been found valuable.

A special effort has been made to produce good color illustrations of those disease processes which can be suspected or diagnosed from C.S.F. cell preparations. The atlas is not meant to be a textbook of neurology or general pathological anatomy, nor a book on the history of examination of the C.S.F. It is intended to be a practical manual for the worker behind the microscope. Accordingly, there is no discussion of nonspecific changes in the C.S.F. associated with tumors, such as protein elevation, decreased sugar content, pleiocytosis etc. Such data are circumstantial evidence, but in general they prove nothing and they may be the cause of serious mistakes. Tumor cells may be present in C.S.F. despite a normal cell count and a normal protein level.

There is discussion of the cell yield and of certain staining methods, as well as of the morphological characteristics of cells in:

a) normal C.S.F. (including incidental findings);
b) traumatic processes and hemorrhage;
c) bacterial and viral diseases;
d) tumor cells in the C.S.F.

Chapter 2

Normal and abnormal C.S.F.: General remarks
(Fig. 2-1–Fig. 2-16)

In normal C.S.F. only lymphocytes and monocytes are found. The nuclei of lymphocytes and monocytes are often more polymorphic than in blood smears. Sayk suggested the very useful term 'lymphoid and monocytoid cells'. Plasma cells, too, show similar polymorphism; hence names like 'immature plasma cells', 'activated plasma cells' and 'plasmacytoid cells' are in use. Neutrophil cells look the same as in blood smears.

Now and then, however, small sheets of tissue of no significance may be observed in C.S.F. from patients with, for example, a disc prolapse. They may be fragments of pia, arachnoid, ependyma or choroid plexus. Similar clusters of cells are more often found in head trauma, hemorrhage, infectious diseases and tumors. They are also very common in all forms of hydrocephalus. These tissue fragments which have no diagnostic significance can easily be mistaken by the beginner for clumps of tumor cells. Arachnoid tissue which for unknown reasons often shows nuclear polymorphism is especially likely to lead to false positive (tumor) findings.

Tissue fragments of pia are characterized by basophil cytoplasm and widely dispersed small, round or oval nuclei (Fig. 2-1–Fig. 2-4). Arachnoid tissue has cells with light or dark blue color and round or oval nuclei. The nuclei may be crowded or relatively widely dispersed (Fig. 2-5–Fig. 2-8). Tissue fragments of ependymal cells show a mauve, light pink or light blue-colored cytoplasm. The nuclei are typically round or slightly oval, and they are hyperchromatic (Fig. 2-9–Fig. 2-12). Choroid plexus cells have a mauve-colored or light pink cytoplasm, which is often finely granulated. The nuclei are not hyperchromatic (Fig. 2-13–Fig. 2-16). Sometimes clumps of cells show a combination of the characteristics of ependyma and choroid plexus in which case differentiation is impossible. Choroid plexus cells, however, are PAS-positive, but ependyma cells are not (Rubinstein 1972; Oehmichen 1976).

Neutrophils in the C.S.F. are always a pathological finding. They occur in hemorrhage, thrombotic and infectious processes and in cases of tumor (Fig. 4a-1–Fig. 4a-2).

Eosinophil granulocytes (Fig. 3-4) are always a pathological finding. They occur in small numbers in all circumstances in which neutrophil granulocytes are found. They are seen in larger numbers in parasitic diseases of the C.N.S., in cases with foreign bodies (drains!), allergic processes, intrathecal penicillin, after myelography and in malignant lymphomas.

Plasma cells are always pathological. They are found especially in viral diseases, in the recovery phase of bacterial meningitis, in multiple sclerosis and in luetic infection. Their characteristics are cytoplasm with an azure (corn flower) color, a round, eccentric nucleus and a perinuclear halo.

For unknown reasons the classic wheel-spike nuclear chromatin structure is almost always absent from cells in the C.S.F. Very often immature plasma cells are seen with a larger nucleus and darker staining cytoplasm. The significance of plasma cells in the C.S.F. has been extensively discussed by Greger and Wieczorek (1966) (Fig. 4a-6–Fig. 4a-7). Spriggs (1954) described myeloma cells in the C.S.F. in a case of plasmocytoma.

The presence of eosinophil or neutrophil granulocytes in the C.S.F. has been regarded by some authors as an argument against multiple sclerosis. Erythrocytes may be present as an artefact after inexpert spinal puncture, and in all cases of head trauma, arachnoid hemorrhage and tumor. When the erythrocytes have a normal configuration, as in blood smears, the hemorrhage is an artefact (or fresh). As the erythrocytes become older they appear washed-out and stain poorly. The presence of macrophages phagocytozing erythrocytes shows that the red blood cells have been in the C.S.F. for at least a few hours (Fig. 3-1–Fig. 3-3).

Macrophages or histiocytes are altered monocytes according to some authors, and altered arachnoid cells according to others. As there are often macrophages in tissue fragments, at least those cells must be of arachnoidal origin (Fig. 3-3).
Macrophages may contain black pigment, especially in instances of old hemorrhage (hemosiderin). Yellow pigment is rarely found; it is hematoidin.

Cartilage cells can be found after an inexpert lumbar puncture. They have burgundy-colored, granular cytoplasm, distinct cell borders and dark red-violet nuclei (Fig. 3-5).

The most important pathological finding is the presence of sheets of tumor cells. The major part of this atlas is concerned with the diagnosis of tumors. Specific problems of tumors are discussed in Chapters 6, 7 and 8.

Chapter 3

Traumatic processes and hemorrhages
(Fig. 3-1–Fig. 3-3)

A bloody spinal tap is a very important finding. The first question to be asked then is whether the blood-staining is an artefact. Direct centrifugation of the spinal fluid will show slight or strong xanthochromia of the supernatant after spontaneous hemorrhage or head trauma, provided that the puncture is done at least 6 hours after the accident.

A colorless supernatant is found when the admixture of blood has been caused by a clumsy spinal puncture. In that case almost nothing except fresh erythrocytes is seen in the C.S.F. cell slide and there will be only a few white blood cells. When a bloody spinal fluid is examined a few hours after a spontaneous hemorrhage or head trauma, the same cytological picture is seen. If the hemorrhage is older, however, macrophages can be seen phagocytozing erythrocytes (Fig. 3-3).

After some time there may be a reaction, with the appearance of all kinds of white blood cells (lymphocytes, monocytes, neutrophil granulocytes, eosinophil granulocytes and plasma cells). The neutrophil leucocyte reaction can be so strong that the diagnosis of meningitis must be considered. In cases of head trauma with nasal liquorrhea or otorrhea the combination of bloody spinal fluid and bacterial meningitis is possible.

After a hemorrhagic infarct of the brain, for example, a sterile reaction in the leptomeninges can be the cause of admixture of erythrocytes and neutrophil leucocytes. Differentiation by cytological means is then impossible, and the clinical picture, examination of a Gram-stained preparation and bacteriological examination are required to make the diagnosis.

When spinal taps are repeated, all cytological characteristics become less pronounced. When the patient recovers from head trauma or spontaneous hemorrhage (arachnoid hemorrhage etc.), the spinal fluid clears up and again becomes normal. If there is recurrent bleeding, the signs of old and fresh hemorrhages are present, and macrophages with black pigment (hemosiderin), or more rarely yellow pigment (hematoidin) are found.

Similar types of macrophages are also seen in cases of birth trauma, hydrocephalus and after neurosurgical operations.

Bacterial and viral diseases
(Fig. 4a-1–Fig. 4a-7)

Diagnosis of bacterial meningitis is greatly facilitated by a C.S.F. cell preparation. The typical picture is that of innumerable neutrophil granulocytes with an occasional lymphocyte or monocyte (Fig. 4a-1–Fig. 4a-2). Examination by Gram staining should reveal gram-positive or gram-negative bacteria, especially the most frequently found *Diplococcus pneumoniae, Neisseria meningitidis* and *Haemophilus influenzae* (Fig. 4a-3–Fig. 4a-4). Tuberculous meningitis from the start shows a higher percentage of lymphocytes and monocytes than of neutrophils. Rarely is it possible, with Ziehl–Neelsen staining, to find a tubercle bacillus.

Using the Gram preparation, *Cryptococcus neoformans* can also be found (Fig. 4a-5).

The further course of the bacterial meningitis can be followed in succesive C.S.F. cell slides. In the recovery phase a decrease of neutrophil granulocytes and an increase in lymphocytes, monocytes and later of plasma cells is found. There is a simultaneous decrease in the total cell count per μl of C.S.F. If the patient does not recover with treatment the total number of cells again increases and the cytological picture shows a shift toward an increased number of neutrophil granulocytes. Small numbers of eosinophils may be present in all phases of bacterial meningitis. In some cases very large numbers of eosinophil granulocytes are found. This can be due to the presence of a foreign body (Spitz–Holter or other neurosurgical draining procedures), or by parasitic infection (mostly in tropical countries, cysticercosis etc.), or to an allergic reaction (intrathecal penicillin, myelography and pneumo-encephalography) (Fig. 3-4).

Lymphocytic meningitis in the majority of cases is caused by a viral infection, but this can never be proven by a routine cytological examination. The specific diagnosis of certain viruses in cytological preparations is now possible by use of immunofluorescence techniques (see Chapter 4b).

A characteristic of viral meningitis is the presence of very many lymphocytes and monocytes and only a low percentage of neutrophil granulocytes. After 5–7 days almost all granulocytes have disappeared. Later on plasma cells are found in increasing numbers, including immature forms (they have a larger cell body and nucleus and darker cytoplasm), (Fig. 4a-6–Fig. 4a-7).

Tuberculous meningitis can show a great similarity to viral lymphocytic meningitis, but only in the later phases and in untreated cases. Luetic disease, multiple sclerosis and brain abscesses can have the characteristics of a lymphocytic meningitis, but the total cell count is usually lower than in viral infections. In multiple sclerosis total cell counts exceeding $300/\mu$l are very rare.

C.S.F. cell immunofluorescence in viral neurological disease

(Fig. 4b-1–Fig. 4b-9)

Application of immunofluorescence (IF) to C.S.F. cells to identify viral antigens may establish a viral diagnosis at the earliest opportunity. However, the reported data and the types of virus investigated are limited. In particular, the procedure has still to be put into perspective with respect to HSV encephalitis.

Some comments on the C.S.F. cell IF technique (Dayan and Stokes 1972; Peters 1979) are required.

In general, the reliability of IF procedures is critically dependent on the quality of the reagents and on the control methods for specificity of the reaction. In fact, if IF is used for diagnosis of viral infection 'the ultimate and absolute control' (Gardner and MacQuillin 1974) is isolation of the virus by standard culture methods from specimens which show positive fluorescence.

A prerequisite for successful IF staining is the preparation of C.S.F. slides with as many cells as possible in as good a condition. Time delay between lumbar puncture and preparation of slides must be minimised.

Knowledge of and experience with the various appearances of fluorescent cells in infected tissue cultures is of major importance; for example, cytoplasmic fluorescence together with rounding of cells and an eccentric nucleus in enterovirus-infected C.S.F. cells (Fig. 4b-3) strikingly resembles the pattern observed in enterovirus-infected tissue cultures.

In the majority of cases it is the mononuclear cells in C.S.F. that show IF staining, but occasionally polymorphonuclear leukocytes may be stained (Fig. 4b-5).

All authors report a low percentage of fluorescent cells per slide, thus underlining the desirability of examining as many slides as possible.

Nonspecific IF or autofluorescence of cells does not cause major problems in deciding whether an IF test is positive or negative.

The following table summarizes certain aspects of positive results (reported in the literature and personal experience) of C.S.F. cell immunofluorescence in neurological disease of viral origin.

Table 4b-1. Positive results of C.S.F. cell immunofluorescence for viral antigens.

Clinical entity	Viral antigen identified	Localisation of fluorescence	References
Encephalitis; meningitis	Herpes simplex	intranuclear/ intranuclear and cytoplasmic/ cytoplasmic	Sommerville (1966); Marshall (1967); Dayan and Stokes (1972); Jarrat and Hubler (1974); Taber et al. (1976); Peters (1979).
Cerebellar ataxia; nervous system complications of herpes zoster	Varicella-zoster	intranuclear/ intranuclear and cytoplasmic	Shoji et al. (1976); Peters et al. (1978a, 1979a).
Meningitis; encephalitis	Mumps	cytoplasmic	Sommerville (1966); Boyd and Vince-Ribaric (1973); Peters (1979).
Meningoencephalitis; cerebellar ataxia; hemichorea; facial nerve palsy; paralytic poliomyelitis	ECHO, Coxsackie A and B (different types); Polio I	cytoplasmic	Sommerville (1966); Taber et al. (1973); Peters (1979); Peters et al. (1978b, 1979b).
Congenital rubella	Rubella	cytoplasmic	Peters and Versteeg
Subacute sclerosing panencephalitis (SSPE)	Measles	cytoplasmic	Dayan and Stokes (1971, 1972); Lindeman et al. (1974); Peters (1979).
Progressive multifocal leukoencephalopathy (PML)	SV40	intranuclear	Peters et al. (1979c)

Chapter 5

Tumors: General remarks

The finding of tumor cells in the C.S.F. is of the utmost importance. There are, however, many misunderstandings by neurologists, neurosurgeons and other specialists of the significance of examination of C.S.F. for tumor cells. They can be found only when the tumor has reached the C.S.F. compartment! If this has not occurred, a large intracerebral tumor may still be present despite a negative C.S.F. preparation.

In the literature very different percentages of the frequency of positive findings have been reported. The differences are caused by the following factors:

1) Type of specimen used: ventricular, suboccipital or spinal fluid. The percentage of positive findings in the ventricular fluid is much higher than in spinal fluid.
2) How often the C.S.F. is examined: Sometimes, in a series of spinal taps only one is positive, or only one of two or three preparations made from the same C.S.F. is positive.
3) Whether the C.S.F. is examined before or after an operation: A pre-operative spinal tap can be negative, whereas after the operation it is positive. This has been found particularly in meningiomas and a neuroma.
4) The experience of the cytologist: This is the problem of the 'false' negative and 'false' positive.

   A patient with a tumor that has not reached the C.S.F. compartment will have a C.S.F. without tumor cells. This, however, is not a 'false' negative, but a case in which tumor cells have been unable to reach the C.S.F. Possibly at a later date the C.S.F. may become positive for tumor cells (or not!). For the same reason all extradural tumors are invariably 'negative' in the C.S.F. Meningiomas very rarely exfoliate and neurinomas do so extremely rarely in the C.S.F.

   A 'false' negative can also mean that tumor cells, or clusters of tumor cells, have been erroneously considered to be arachnoid tissue, or that small solitary tumor cells have been called lymphocytes or monocytes, for example, in cases of oat cell carcinoma or neuroblastoma.

   'False positive' represents the contrary phenomenon. Arachnoid tissue may have an activated appearance. The nuclei may be rather crowded and polymorphic. The author often made this mistake in the beginning. Cases of hydrocephalus are well known for often showing cells suspicious of a tumor and tumor fragments even when no tumor is present.

In other cases tumor cells may be found when the clinician has not diagnosed a tumor. This occurred especially in the period before the C.T. scan was introduced. When the patient returned after some while the presence of a tumor would be confirmed. The so-called 'false' positive had been the only positive sign of the tumor.

5) The types of patients are different:

Is the tumor percentage reported from a cancer institute or from a general hospital, or from a neurological department, or from a neurosurgical department?

Is the percentage based on the total number of all spinal fluids (inclusive of well diagnosed disc prolapse and meningitis cases) or only from cases suspected of or diagnosed as having a tumor. Thus, a simple statement of the percentage of positive diagnosis of tumors is meaningless; in the literature percentages of 3% to 51% are mentioned.

In the cytopathology of C.S.F. the examiner of the specimen lacks evidence of invasion and architectural disarray. Furthermore the hypotonic C.S.F. causes distortion of the cells by making them swell and its enzymes may produce autolysis. This may be contrasted with staining in pathology, which is mostly done with hematoxylin-eosin on paraffin sections of formalin-fixed material. Paraffin sections cause considerable shrinkage of the tissue and C.S.F. causes swelling.

In cytology staining is mostly done with the May–Grünwald–Giemsa, the Jenner–Giemsa, or the Papanicolaou techniques, which give entirely different appearances from that of hematoxylin-eosin staining (Fig. 6-3-8).

For teaching, training and comparison, paraffin sections are useless. The best materials for study are smear preparations made from fresh surgical specimens or from unfixed autopsy material, stained with one of the cytological staining techniques (McCormick and Coleman, 1962).

Aspirates of tumor cysts treated in the same way as C.S.F. cell slides are also very useful, because cells and clusters of cells often have the same morphology and staining qualities as tumor cells. Cyst contents often show marked autolysis.

What are the distinguishing features or characteristics of tumor cells? Many points are mentioned in the literature but most important are:

1) anisokaryosis;
2) anisocytosis;
3) large nuclei;
4) large cells (sometimes giant cells) or very small cells;

    } variation in size and shape of cells and nuclei

5) the nucleus–cell ratio is increased in favor of the nucleus;
6) irregular nuclear margins;
7) prominent, enlarged and multiple nucleoli, often hyperchromatic;

8) marked hyperchromasia and clumping of chromatin, metachromasia and polychromasia;
9) mitoses in clusters of cells and abnormal mitoses (mitosis of free-lying cells may also be seen in nontumorous diseases, for example in bacterial meningitis).

Features 1–9 produce the strong impression of pleomorphism, but none is pathognomonic of a tumor. When, however, there is a series of positive tumor characteristics the diagnosis becomes certain. Papanicolaou gives a gradation in five groups, but for practical purposes we prefer:

1) no tumor cells are present;
2) suspicious cells are present, but tumor diagnosis is not proven;
3) positive for tumor cells; if possible, a more specific diagnosis is given.

Class 1 does not exclude a tumor, as described above under 'false' negative. Class 2 means, beware: further diagnostic examinations are necessary; class 3, there is a tumor whatever the opinion of the clinician.

A specific diagnosis should be possible in a proportion of the cases. The differential diagnosis may be possible between primary tumors and metastatic tumors. In favorable cases of primary tumors, astrocytomas, medulloblastomas, ependymomas and oligodendrogliomas may be distinguished. In cases of metastatic tumor the differential diagnosis between squamous cell carcinoma, adenocarcinoma and undifferentiated tumor is possible. Melanoma, when not amelanotic, can be recognized.

Chapter 6

Primary tumors of the C.N.S.

6-1 Astrocytoma (Fig. 6-1-1–Fig. 6-1-34)
They were placed by Kernohan and Sayre in Grades I–IV, of which Grade I is the least and Grade IV the most malignant.

Grade I (Fig. 6-1-1–Fig. 6-1-4)
Grade I astrocytoma is often very difficult to recognize. There is a small increase of the number and the nuclei are a little larger than normal.

Grade II (Fig. 6-1-5–Fig. 6-1-13)
There is some more crowding, pleomorphism and anisokaryosis of the nuclei.

Grade III (Fig. 6-1-14–Fig. 6-1-23)
Definite pleomorphism and variation in the size and shape of the nuclei is seen and pronounced hyperchromasia is present. There are mitoses and tumor giant cells.

Grade IV (Fig. 6-1-24–Fig. 6-1-34)
There are nuclei of all sorts of shape and size, and there are many mitoses and giant tumor cells. These tumors are identical with glioblastoma multiforme.

Areas of different grades of malignancy can be found in a tumor and the same holds true for the tissue fragments and single tumor cells in C.S.F.

Bots et al. (1964) described that low grade astrocytoma cells have eosinophilic cytoplasm with ill-defined cellular margins. In grade III and IV astrocytomas the cytoplasm is basophilic and the cellular outline is well defined.

Bischof (1961) and Naylor (1961) held that primary and metastatic tumors can be differentiated in the C.S.F. Differential diagnosis between a primary and metastatic tumor may be impossible in some cases.

6-2 Medulloblastoma (Fig. 6-2-1–Fig. 6-2-8)
These tumors arise from the cells of the external granular layer of the cerebellum. This opinion is not accepted by all authors.

Tissue sheets of medulloblastoma show pronounced cellular pleomorphism. Sometimes there is extreme crowding of nuclei, scanty cytoplasm and the nuclei may almost fill the entire cell body. Pseudorosettes may be present. Whorls and palisades are also described. Neuronal maturation toward ganglion cells is rare. Mitoses can very often be found in tissue fragments. In other fragments there may be far less crowding and pronounced pleochromatism of the cytoplasm.

Medulloblastoma and retinoblastoma show a close resemblance and differentiation on cytopathological criteria is not always possible. Retinoblastoma is much rarer than medulloblastoma. Stefanko (1972) and Kölmel (1976), respectively, have published good black and white and color photographs of medulloblastoma cells in the C.S.F.

6-3 Ependymoma (Fig. 6-3-1—Fig. 6-3-8)

Ependymomas are tumors arising from the ependyma, so they are in direct contact with the C.S.F. It is astonishing therefore, that tumor cells are relatively rarely found in C.S.F. preparations. The tumor cells closely resemble ependyma. There is, however, anisokaryosis, pleomorphism, and hyperchromatism, which makes it possible to differentiate them from normal ependyma: the more outspoken the pleomorphism the more malignant the tumor. Sometimes rosette formation of tumor cells can be seen in C.S.F. cell preparations. They have the same morphology and staining qualities as smear preparations of fresh ependymoma stained with the Jenner—Giemsa technique (Fig. 2-9).

6-4 Oligodendroglioma (Fig. 6-4-1—Fig. 6-4-9)

These are tumors arising from oligodendroglia.

The nuclei are sometimes crowded and sometimes more widely dispersed. Anisokaryosis is not pronounced, which gives the examiner the impression of only modest pleomorphism. In histological preparations a clear halo around the nuclei is often found, but in C.S.F. preparations the halo is usually absent. The halo in the histological preparation may be an artefact of autolysis, or it may be the result from fixation of the tissue. Oligodendroglial cells may be strongly PAS-positive.

6-5 Pinealoma (Fig. 6-5-1—Fig. 6-5-6)

Several different types of tumor occur in the pineal region, including teratomas, germinomas (atypical teratoma or pinealoma), pineablastoma and pineacytoma (Russell and Rubinstein 1971).

McCormick and Coleman (1962) described a large clump of cells from a patient with a 'pinealoma', in which two types of cells were seen. One type was formed by small lymphocyte-like cells and the other consisted of large epithelioid cells. The tumor was a germinoma (the atypical teratoma or pinealoma of Russell and Rubinstein) (Fig. 6-5-1—Fig. 6-5-6).

6-6 Choroid plexus papilloma (Fig. 6-6-1–Fig. 6-6-3)
The papilloma originates from the choroid plexus and has more or less the same structure, consisting of a single layer of epithelium upon a stroma of connective tissue (Fig. 6-6-1). The malignant type is a carcinoma.

6-7 Chromophobe adenoma (Fig. 6-7-1–Fig. 6-7-5)

6-8 Eosinophil adenoma (Fig. 6-8-1–Fig. 6-8-2)
Chromophobe adenomas (some of them prolactinomas) are pituitary tumors with cells that lack granules and have no particular tinctorial affinity.

Eosinophil adenomas are pituitary tumors the cells of which contain eosinophilic granules.

This conventional nomenclature is obsolete. In any case, in a C.S.F. preparation the distinction cannot be made between a chromophobe and an eosinophil tumor.

The color photographs show a cyst aspirate and a smear preparation from a patient with a chromophobe adenoma, and a C.S.F. preparation from another patient. The nuclei are round and hyperchromatic. The cell borders are well defined.

A cyst aspirate from a patient with an eosinophil adenoma is also illustrated. A C.S.F. cell slide from an eosinophil adenoma was not available in our series.

6-9 Craniopharyngeoma (Fig. 6-9-1–Fig. 6-9-5)
They are derived from Rathke's pouch, a remnant of the craniopharyngeal canal, and have an epithelial structure. The tissue sheets are made up of stratified, epidermoid epithelium and palisaded epithelial cells.

Cell nests and palisading can be recognized in cyst puncture preparations from craniopharyngiomas.

Cholesterol crystals may also be found in these preparations.

6-10 Meningioma (Fig. 6-10-1–Fig. 6-10-10)
This tumor arises from arachnoid cells.

Fibroblastic meningiomas consist of elongated fusiform cells. Whorls may be recognizable in C.S.F. cell preparations. The endotheliomatous type has cells, which often bear a great resemblance to arachnoid cells. Although a meningioma is a benign tumor, there is anisokaryosis and hyperchromasia. The nuclei are often larger than those of arachnoid cells and are more polymorphic in size and shape. In this type, too, a kind of whorling pattern can sometimes be seen. Wilkins and Odom (1966) published a photograph of a cluster of meningioma cells.

6-11 Neurinoma (Neuroma, Schwannoma) (Fig. 6-11-1−Fig. 6-11-3)
They arise mostly from the acoustic nerve in the cerebellopontine angle. They are derived from Schwann cells. All authors are of the opinion that tumor fragments or cells of neuroma are never found in the C.S.F.

In this atlas, however, photographs are presented from a case after operation, in whom there was extensive spread of tissue sheets and cells in the C.S.F., even in the lumbar space. The histological pattern consists of bundles of fibers and spindle cells, and whorls or palisading can be seen. The differential diagnosis from fibroblastic meningioma is difficult.

6-12 Colloid cyst (Fig. 6-12-1)
According to some authors these cysts are derived from ependyma, but others consider that they arise from the choroid plexus. The C.S.F. preparation from one case probably shows part of the lining of a colloid cyst. The nuclei have more pleomorphism than was expected in this 'benign' disease.

Chapter 7

Metastatic tumors in the C.N.S.

In the literature there is disagreement about the feasibility of differential diagnosis between primary tumors and metastatic tumors of the C.N.S.

The difference of opinion has arisen from consideration of two very large groups of tumors, each of which embraces many types of neoplasm of very different morphology. The lower grade astrocytomas have a light pink cytoplasm and ill-defined cell margins. Metastatic adenocarcinomas of the respiratory and intestinal tracts have cells with basophilic cytoplasm and well-defined margins.

Astrocytomas Grade III and IV, however, have mauve or light blue-staining cytoplasm and well-defined cell margins, and so do pinealomas and pituitary tumors. It will be apparent, therefore, that generalisations cannot be made.

7-1 Squamous carcinoma of the lung (Fig. 7-1-1–Fig. 7-1-10)
The most frequent tumor of the lung is the bronchogenic carcinoma. It is divided into squamous cell carcinoma, adenocarcinoma and undifferentiated carcinoma of large or small cell pattern.

Other types are rare and will not be discussed, because we have no experience of them in C.S.F. preparations. Squamous cell carcinoma is characterized by a bluish opaque or pale violet cytoplasm. This can be seen after Jenner–Giemsa staining. In the Papanicolaou stain the cells have a bright orange color. Light blue granules in the cytoplasm can be seen with the Jenner–Giemsa stain. There are also anaplastic types containing small or large cells, in which case diagnosis of the primary tumor is not possible.

7-2 Adenocarcinoma of the lung (Fig. 7-2-1–Fig. 7-2-4)
Adenocarcinoma of the lung may contain mucinous secretion, which can be demonstrated by PAS-staining. Signet ring cells may be present. The oat cell carcinoma is the anaplastic, small cell type.

7-3 Carcinoma of the breast (Fig. 7-3-1–Fig. 7-3-8)
The majority of breast cancers arise in the ductal epithelium. They are mostly adenocarcinomas and may or may not contain mucin (mucinous carcinoma,

positive PAS-stain). Signet ring cells may be present, which contain large vacuoles of mucin. Sometimes glandular or papillary structures may be seen in tissue fragments in the C.S.F. (medullary adenocarcinoma) (Fig. 7-3-8). The cells often show poor adhesion and therefore lie singly, sometimes in great numbers, in the C.S.F. cell preparation.

In some cases the number of tumor cells may be so large that meningitis carcinomatosa can be diagnosed.

7-4 *Carcinoma of the stomach* (Fig. 7-4-1—Fig. 7-4-8)

The histologic pattern is that of an adenocarcinoma. Signet ring cells containing mucin are often present. Carcinoma of the stomach is often the cause of meningitis carcinomatosa.

Their diagnosis will become more important in the future when chemotherapy is more advanced.

7-5 *Carcinoma of the colon* (Fig. 7-5-1—Fig. 7-5-2)

The majority of cancers of the colon are adenocarcinomas. Dedifferentiation may be observed.

7-6 *Carcinoma of the rectum* (Fig. 7-6-1—Fig. 7-6-4)

The histological appearance of carcinoma of the rectum is identical with that of adenocarcinoma of the colon.

7-7 *Carcinoma of the pancreas* (Fig. 7-7-1—Fig. 7-7-3)

The majority of carcinomas of the pancreas are adenocarcinoma. They show a glandular pattern and may or may not secrete mucin. Dedifferentiation can occur.

7-8 *Melanoma* (Fig. 7-8-1—Fig. 7-8-8)

Melanomas arise from melanin producing cells. In the past these tumors were called melanosarcoma, as they were thought to have a mesodermal origin. The present opinion is that they originate from ectoderm and should be called melanocarcinoma. However, the most common name is melanoma (Robbins 1974).

Cases which come to a neurological clinic usually have a neoplasm of a very malignant type.

The cytological characteristics are those of any carcinoma, but the diagnosis can be made by the presence of melanin pigment in the tumor cells.

The tumor cells may be nonpigmented, in which case staining with the DOPA or Schmorl's reaction may make it possible to reach the correct diagnosis. The Schmorl stain can be done on a fixed preparation, but the DOPA stain has to be done on an unfixed, unstained preparation.

7-9 Retinoblastoma (Fig. 7-9-1–Fig. 7-9-4)
These tumors are neuroblastomas developing in the retina. Cytoplasm is scanty and the cell groups are very compact. Mitoses are frequent. Giant cells are absent. It may be difficult or impossible to differentiate a retinoblastoma from a medulloblastoma on cytological grounds alone.

7-10 Neuroblastoma (Fig. 7-10-1–Fig. 7-10-4)
This tumor arises from an adrenal gland or from the sympathetic chain. The cells are small and dark, like lymphocytes.

Chapter 8

Malignant lymphoma and hemoblastoma involving the C.N.S.

8-1 Reticulosarcoma, lymphosarcoma or non-Hodgkin lymphoma
Malignant lymphomas were previously divided into lymphosarcoma and reticulosarcoma. Lymphosarcoma was the term applied to proliferation of cells like small lymphocytes and reticulosarcoma represented proliferation of cells of more variable type (Fig. 8-1-1–Fig. 8-1-4).

This nomenclature was modified by Rappaport (1969), and subsequently by the classification of Lennert and Lukes. At present all classifications are temporary and there is not yet a uniform nomenclature for malignant lymphomas.

Malignant lymphomas may be nodular or diffuse. They do not arise from reticulum cells but from lymphocytes. If there is immunological differentiation T and B cell lymphomas can be distinguished.

In all cases in which C.S.F. was presented for examination the terminology of the clinician and pathologist has been used in the legends of the color photographs (Fig. 8-1-5–Fig. 8-1-10).

8-2 Lymphoblastic leukemia (Fig. 8-2-1–Fig. 8-2-2)

8-3 Myeloblastic leukemia (Fig. 8-3-1–Fig. 8-3-2)
Examination of the C.S.F. in hemoblastomas (leukemias) is of considerable interest for two reasons; first, to make the diagnosis of meningeal involvement, and second for follow-up of the results of intrathecal cytostatic therapy. It is important that meningeal involvement may be found before there are leukemic cells in the blood smear.

If no C.S.F. cell preparation has been made, examination solely by means of the counting chamber may give the false impression of a lymphocytic meningitis.

The morphology of the diverse types of leukemic cells in the C.S.F. is the same as in the corresponding peripheral blood smears.

Miscellaneous Conditions

Case for diagnosis (Fig. 10-1-1).
The patient, a 2-month-old boy, developed hydrocephalus. Toxoplasmosis tests

were negative. At pneumoencephalography occlusion of the foramen of Monro was found. The C.S.F. contained macrophages. These cells had phagocytized plasma cells. The spinal fluid contained also a considerable number of neutrophils, lymphocytes and monocytes. The etiology of this case was undetermined. Phagocytosis of plasma cells is a very unusual phenomenon.

Case for diagnosis (Fig. 10-1-2).
The patient, a 61-year-old man, had a history of Addison's disease. On admission to hospital he was sleepy, and there was meningeal irritation and papiloedema. In the spinal fluid many tissue fragments and single cells were found with all the characteristics of tumor cells. X-ray pictures of the lung were normal. Examination of the sputum for tumor cells was negative on three occasions. The condition of the patient deteriorated rapidly. A few days after admission he died. Autopsy was refused by the family.

C.S.F. cell preparation: the cytoplasm of the tumor cells resembles that of squamous carcinoma cells but the primary tumor is not identified.

An electron micrograph of the virus of infectious mononucleosis is presented in Plate 1-1. It is an as yet unpublished observation by the author.

Chapter 9

Methods for the preparation of C.S.F. cells

In the introduction, the three major techniques for preparation of C.S.F. cells were mentioned. They are:

a) the sedimentation method (after Sayk);
b) the Millipore or Nucleopore filter methods (membrane filter technique);
c) the centrifugation method.

I prefer the method of Sayk, because the finer details of cells so prepared are best visualized.

The author has had no success with Millipore or Nucleopore methods. There was always considerable shrinkage of the cells and far less detail was seen than with the Sayk method. The most serious criticism of Sayk's method is the large loss of cells.

In 1978, a modification of the Sayk method was published, which gives a high yield of cells. It is described in this chapter.

Those who wish to try the membrane filter or centrifugal methods can find them described in the literature (Kistler and Bischoff 1962; McCormick and Coleman 1962; Metzel 1963; Reynaud and King 1967; Wesemann 1967; Baringer 1970; Kistler 1970; Spaar and Munz 1970; Brucher et al. 1972; Rich 1972; Stokes et al. 1975).

Sayk's technique (Plates 9-1 and 9-2)
The apparatus designed by Sayk consists of a base-plate with a rotating horizontal shaft on which two arms are mounted. These arms carry weights through which a small tube-holder can be fixed (Plate 9-1).

The tube holder contains a small glass cylinder or chamber placed on a filter paper with a round opening of the same diameter as the glass cylinder. A slide is placed below the filter paper. The recommended filter paper is No. 589^3 Best Nr.300202 (Schleicher and Schüll).

When the apparatus is ready for use, C.S.F. (1 ml or less) is placed in the glass cylinder or chamber (Plate 9-2). The filter paper should first be moistened with physiological saline.

The C.S.F. is gradually absorbed by the paper. It is during this absorption that there is loss of about 85% of cells into the filter paper. The duration of the absorption is dependent on the pressure of the weights of the arms. According to these weights the duration of the absorption is about 20–30 minutes. During the sedimentation a number of the cells in the C.S.F. are deposited on the slide. The sediment is then stained according to May–Grünwald–Giemsa or Jenner–Giemsa. I prefer the Jenner–Giemsa method. Other staining techniques may be used (see Chapter 10).

Modified technique

The most modern technique, and possibly the best at present, has been described by Tutuarima, Hische and Van der Helm, of the Laboratory of Clinical Neurochemistry of the Neurological Clinic, University of Amsterdam. It is a modification of the sedimentation method of Sayk. The cytomorphology is as good as that obtained with Sayk's sedimentation technique, but the cell yield is 90%.

The Sayk sedimentation apparatus is used. The cylinder or chamber is a smoothly polished perspex cone with a height of 20mm, an internal diameter at the top of 21mm and at the bottom of 13mm, which is pressed directly on the glass slide by an adjustable lever. This prevents loss of C.S.F. The suction tip is a new variant. It is a disposable 1ml pipette tip (Finn tip nr.61) of which the opening of the point is covered by a Nucleopore filter (pore size 0.4μm, diameter 13mm; Nucleopore Corp., Pleasanton, California).

A piece of double sided Sellotape ($\pm$ 10 $\times$ 3mm) is applied around the point of the disposable tip. The tape projects beyond the top for about 1mm. The adhesive point of the tip is put in the centre of the Nucleopore filter. Next, this filter is folded over the top of the pipette tip. The opening of the pipette is then covered with a filter surface of Nucleopore membrane, because the filter is wrapped around the tip.

The filter is fixed on the tip with a piece of teflon tape (polytetrafluorethylene thread sealing tape). The opening at the top remains free. One third of the tip is filled with Sephadex G10 (paricle size 40–120μm. Pharmacia Fine Chemicals, Sweden). The pipette is placed in the concentration chamber and the tip remains only a small distance above the slide. A clamp fixes the position of the tip.

The C.S.F. fluid is absorbed by the Sephadex particles. The tip and chamber can then be removed and the cells on the slide are ready to be fixed and stained.

The principle is that the tip sucks the fluid from above, instead of from below, as is done by the filter paper in the Sayk method. 0.3ml is sufficient for one cell preparation.

A very simple chamber can be made by glueing a polystyrene tube to a glass slide with chloroform. When the preparation is ready the tube can be removed.

Chapter 10

Staining methods

The simplest and very quick techniques are the May–Grünwald–Giemsa and Jenner–Giemsa stains.

The preparations last for at least 17 years and possibly much longer.

10-1 May–Grünwald–Giemsa fixation and staining
The C.S.F. cells are fixed by pouring 10–15 drops of May–Grünwald solution onto the slide. Stain for 3 minutes. The same volume of water of adjusted pH (7.2) is dripped onto the slide and the mixture allowed to stain for further 2 minutes. Poststaining for 40 minutes is done with a diluted Giemsa solution – 30 drops in water 20ml of pH 7.2. The Giemsa solution must be filtered before use.

10-2 Jenner–Giemsa stain
Fixation for 5 minutes with Jenner solution. The slide is rinsed with tap water and air-dried. Poststaining for 10 minutes with Giemsa solution – 1ml in water 9ml of pH 7.2.

a) May–Grünwald solution.
   May–Grünwald 0.6g + methanol 250ml.
   The solution can be used after 1 week.
   Filter before use.
b) Jenner solution.
   Methylene-blue–eosin Jenner (Ciba) 0.25g + methanol 100ml.
   The solution can be used after 1 week.
   Filter before use.
c) Giemsa solution.
   10 Giemsa tablets + methanol 50ml + glycerol 50ml.
   The solution can be used after 1 week.
   Filter before use.

10-3 Gram stain (for bacteria)
1) Slide air-dried. Short fixation in flame.
2) 1 minute crystal violet solution.

3) Rinse with water.
4) 1 minute lugol solution.
5) Rinse with 96% ethanol.
6) Decolorize 1 minute with 96% ethanol.
7) Rinse with water.
8) 1 minute fuchsin solution.
9) Rinse with water and air-dry the slide.

a) Crystal violet solution: crystal violet 200ml in distilled water 90ml. Add 0.1 M boric acid — borate buffer 10ml (pH 9.0). Prepare this solution fresh every day!
b) Lugol solution. Potassium iodide 2g in distilled water 10ml. Add iodine 1g and add distilled water to 300ml.
c) Fuchsin solution. Fuchsin 200mg in distilled water 100ml.

10-4 Ziehl–Neelsen stain (for Mycobacterium tuberculosis)
1) Carbolic fuchsin 5 minutes on the slide.
   Heat the slide until vapor comes from the fluid.
2) Pour off the carbolic fuchsin.
3) 5% H_2SO_4 for 5 seconds. Shake the slide lightly in the solution.
4) Ethanol 60% for 30 seconds. Shake the slide lightly in the solution.
5) Rinse with tap water.
6) Poststaining with aqueous methylene blue solution for 15 seconds.
7) Rinse with tap water and dry the slide with filterpaper.
Take care not to overstain with the methylene blue.

A
a) Carbolic fuchsin solution. Fuchsin 5g + 96% methanol 95ml.
b) Wait 48 hours. Use a brown bottle. Shake the bottle from time to time.
c) Take 30ml of solution a. Add phenol 18ml.
   Add distilled water to a total volume of 300ml.

B
a) The methylene blue solution is prepared in the same way as in A.a.

10-5 Papanicolaou stain (after Spriggs and Boddington 1968)
 1) Methanol 70% for fixation.
 2) Rinse with distilled water.
 3) Harris hematoxylin for 1 minute.
 4) Rinse with running water; the hematoxylin turns blue.

5) Rinse with methanol 70%.
6) Rinse with methanol 100%.
7) Orange G6 for 1 minute.
8) Rinse with methanol 100%.
9) E.A. 50 for 1 minute.
10) Rinse 4 × with methanol 100%.
11) Xylol for 5 minutes.
12) Mount in DPX.

When membrane filters are used special Papanicolaou stains are prescribed by the manufacturers of the filters.

Papanicolaou staining is not used for routine diagnosis but is valuable in cases of squamous cell carcinoma.

10-6 Sudan black – PAS stain (after De Vries et al.)
1) Fix slide in formaldehyde vapor.
2) Sudan black solution 40 minutes.
3) Rinse with ethanol 70%.
4) Rinse with water
5) Periodic acid 1% for 30 minutes.
6) Rinse 10 minutes with running tap water. Air-dry the slide.
7) Schiff's solution for 45 minutes.
8) Rinse 10 minutes with running tap water.
9) Harris hematoxylin for 15 minutes.
10) Rinse with tap water for 10 minutes.

A
a) Sudan B: 0.5g in 100% ethanol 100ml.
   It takes 48 hours at 37°C to 'ripen' the solution.
b) Phenol 16g in 100% ethanol 30ml.
c) Na_2HPO_4 $12H_2O$ – 0.3g in distilled water 100ml.
Add b. and c.
Take 40ml of the mixture of b. and c. and add 60ml solution a. This mixture must be filtered. It can be used for 2–3 months. Always filter before use.

B Schiff's solution.
a) Para-rosanilin (Merck) 1g in 1N HCl 30ml.
b) Potassium metabisulfite 1g in 170ml distilled water.
Add a. and b. Keep cool at 4°C for 24 hours.
Then clear the solution by adding Norit 600mg. Shake and filter. Keep in brown bottle in the dark at 4°C. The solution can be used for 2 months.

Sudan B–PAS staining is used in cases of leukemia. When the cells are PAS-positive and Sudan black-negative, then the diagnosis is lymphoblastic leukemia. When the cells are strongly Sudan B-positive the diagnosis is myeloblastic leukemia. However, many transitional cases have been observed in which the diagnosis remained doubtful.

10-7 α-naphthyl acetate-esterase stain
1) Fix the slide in formaldehyde vapor for 4.5 minutes at a temperature of 25°C.
2) Rinse with tap water for 5 minutes and air-dry the slide.
3) Incubate with the substrate α-napthyl acetate for 20 minutes at 25°C.
4) Rinse with tap water and air-dry the slide.
5) Stain with Harris hematoxylin for 6 minutes.
6) Rinse with tap water and air-dry the slide.
7) Mount in DPX.

a) α-Naphthyl acetate (Sigma) 20mg in acetone 0.5ml.
b) Add phosphate buffer 20ml – Sörensen (1/15 M, pH 7.4). Shake the mixture.
c) Add fast blue B salt (Gurr) 20mg.

Monoblastic cells show a marked brown granulation. Myeloblasts and lymphoblasts are negative or show only a few brown granules.
   The C.S.F. cell preparations have to be fresh.

10-8 PAS-stain
1) Fix slide in formaldehyde vapor for 5 minutes.
2) Rinse with tap water for 10 minutes.
3) Periodic acid 1% for 30 minutes.
4) Rinse 10 minutes with running tap water. Air-dry the slide.
5) Schiff's solution for 45 minutes.
6) Rinse 10 minutes with running tap water.
7) Harris hematoxylin for 15 minutes.
8) Rinse with tap water for 10 minutes. Air-dry.
For Schiff's solution see under Sudan B–PAS staining.

This technique is used to demonstrate neutral mucopolysaccharides in cases of suspected adenocarcinoma.
a) As fixative 10% formol-methanol (i.e. 40% formaldehyde 10ml + 100% methanol 90ml) can be used instead of formaldehyde vapor.
b) Glycogen is also PAS-positive. Glycogen can be eliminated by incubation in 1% diastase solution for 30 minutes at 37°C.

10-9 Alcian blue stain (for acid mucopolysaccharides)
(after Steedman 1960; cited Pearse 1968).
1) Stain in a freshly filtered 1% solution of Alcian Blue 8GX in 3% acetic acid for
   10–30 minutes.
2) Rinse in distilled water.
3) Stain in 1% neutral red 30 seconds.
4) Dehydrate in alcohol.
5) Clear in xylene.
6) Mount in Canada balsem or DPX.
Results: acid mucopolysaccharides clear blue green, nuclei dark blue or dark red.

In place of Alcian blue 8GX, Alcian green 3BX or Alcian green 2GX can be used.

10-10 Schmorl stain (after Pearse)
1) Stain with ferricyanide solution – 5 minutes (a).
2) Wash in tap water.
3) Stain with 1% neutral red – 3 minutes.
4) Dehydrate in ethanol, xylol and mount in Canada balsem.

a) Ferrycyanide solution is prepared by mixing three parts of 1% ferric chloride or
   ferric sulphate and one part freshly prepared 1% potassium ferricyanide. Use
   within 30 minutes.

Melanin reduces ferricyanide to ferrocyanide (dark blue). Lipofuscin, argentaffin
granules and substances containing active sulphydryl groups also produce a positive
reaction.

10-11 Dopa-oxidase method for melanin
See P. Lopez Cardozo (1975, pg. 649).

10-12 Acid phosphatase stain
See Kaplow and Burstone (1964).

Fig. 2-1 (400 ×)
Patient L. (control case). Smear preparation of pia mater.
The cytoplasm is light blue or light violet.
The nuclei are round or oval and widely dispersed.

Fig. 2-2 (625 ×)
Patient L. (control case). Smear preparation of pia mater.
The cytoplasm is violet. The nuclei round or oval and widely dispersed.

Fig. 2-3 (400 ×)
Patient Y. L.C.S.F. Tissue fragment of pia.

Fig. 2-4 (625 ×)
Patient Y. L.C.S.F. Tissue fragment of pia.

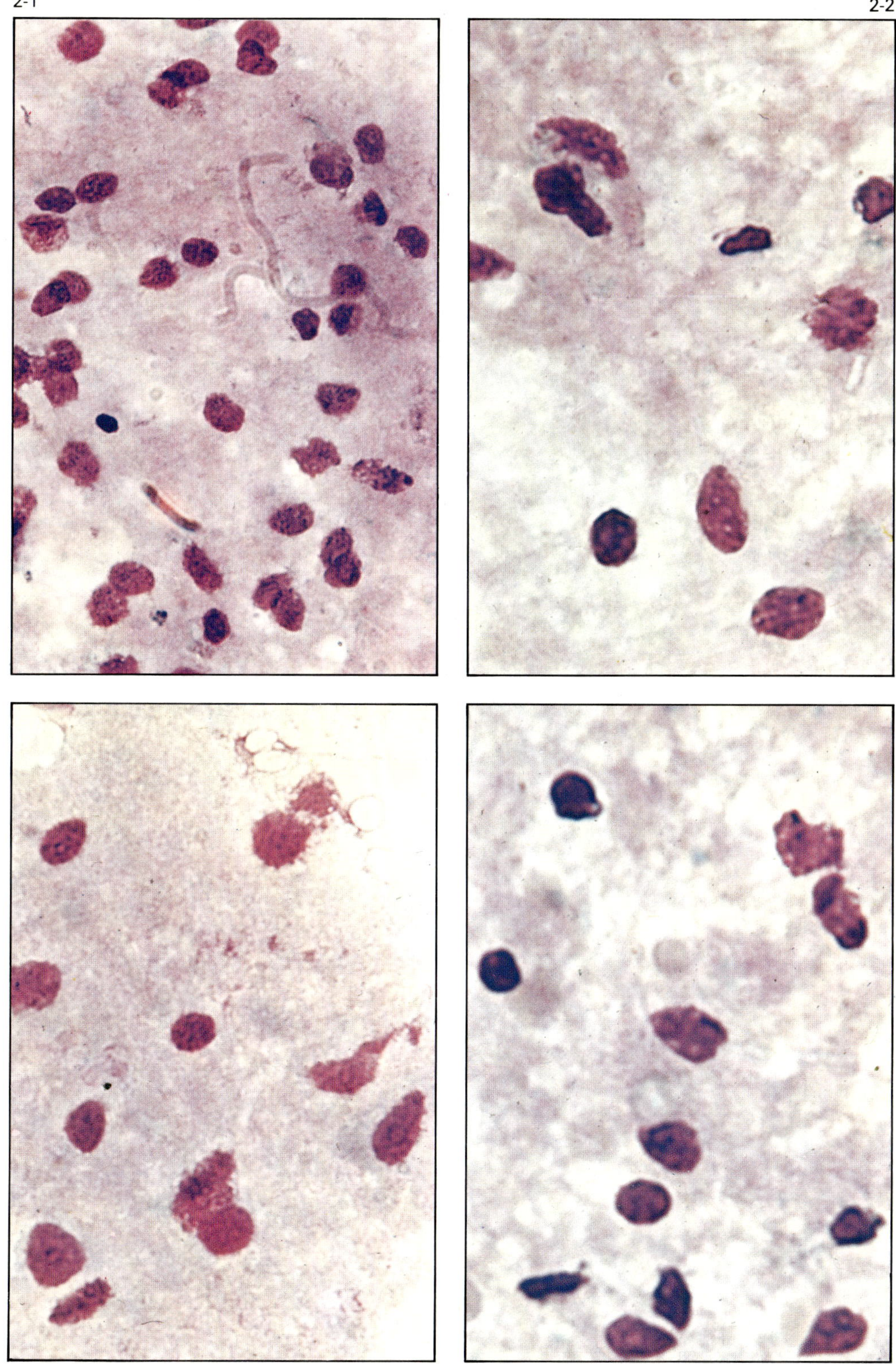
2-1
2-2
2-3
2-4

Fig. 2-5 (625 ×)
Patient W. (control case). Smear preparation of arachnoidea.
The cytological findings can be greatly variable.
Here, the nuclei are oval or have a pronounced elongated shape.

Fig. 2-6 (625 ×)
Patient W. (control case). Smear preparation of arachnoidea.
Marked crowding of round, oval or elongated nuclei.

Fig. 2-7 (625 ×)
Patient d.G. L.C.S.F. Hydrocephalus.
Blue cytoplasm and some variation in shape and size in normal arachnoidea.

Fig. 2-8 (625 ×)
Patient d.G. L.C.S.F. Hydrocephalus. Tissue fragment of arachnoidea.

2-5

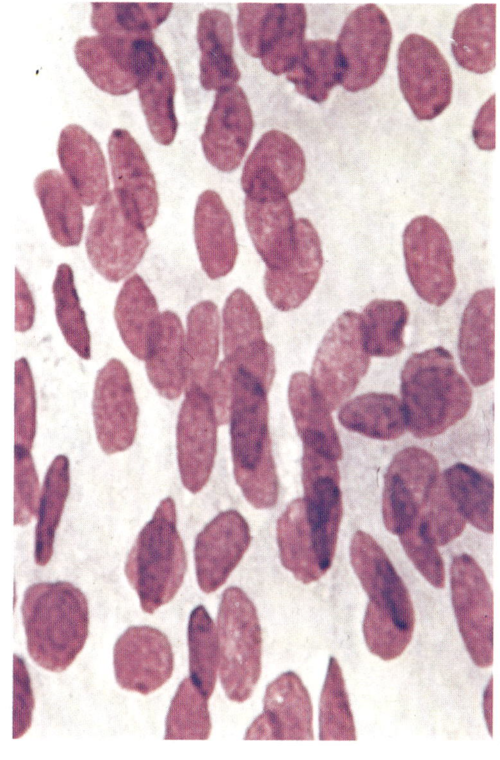

2-6

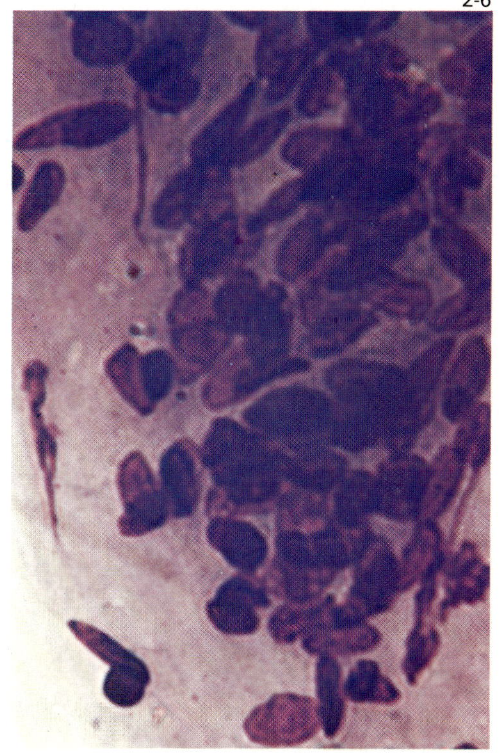

2-7

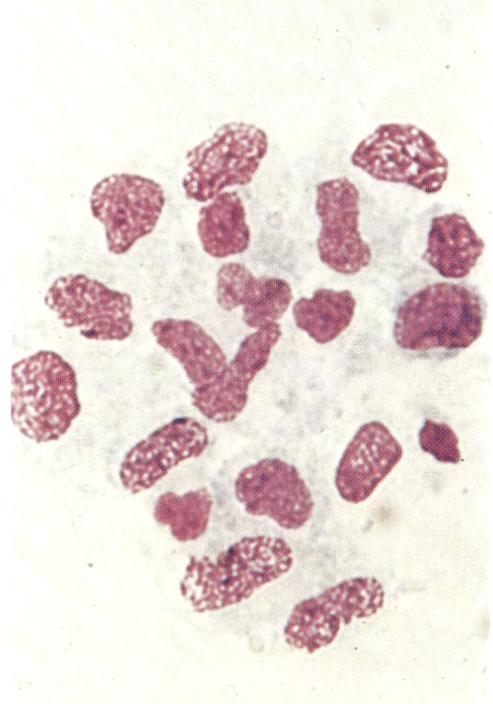

2-8

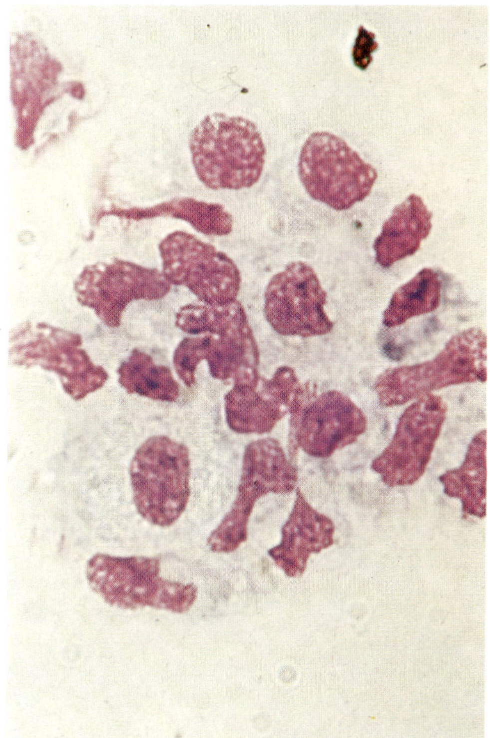

Fig. 2-9 (625×)
Patient H. (control case). Smear preparation of ependyma.
Typical is the hyperchromasia of the nuclei. Some of the nuclei are rounded.

Fig. 2-10 (400×)
Patient H. (control case). Smear preparation of ependyma.
Same characteristics as in fig. 2-9.

Fig. 2-11 (625×)
Patient P. L.C.S.F. Hydrocephalus. Tissue fragment of ependyma cells.
Especially in hydrocephalus cases tissue fragments of pia, arachnoid, plexus and ependyma are found.

Fig. 2-12 (625×)
Patient Ch. L.C.S.F. Hydrocephalus. Tissue fragment of ependyma cells.
Typical are the round hyperchromatic nuclei.

2-9
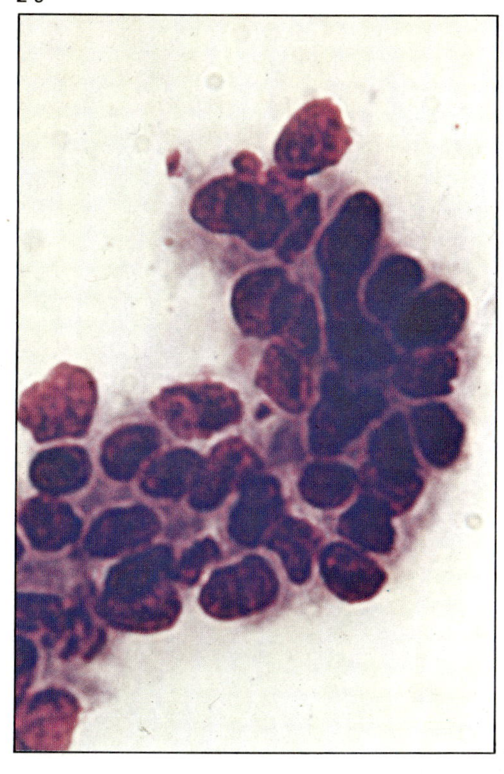

2-10
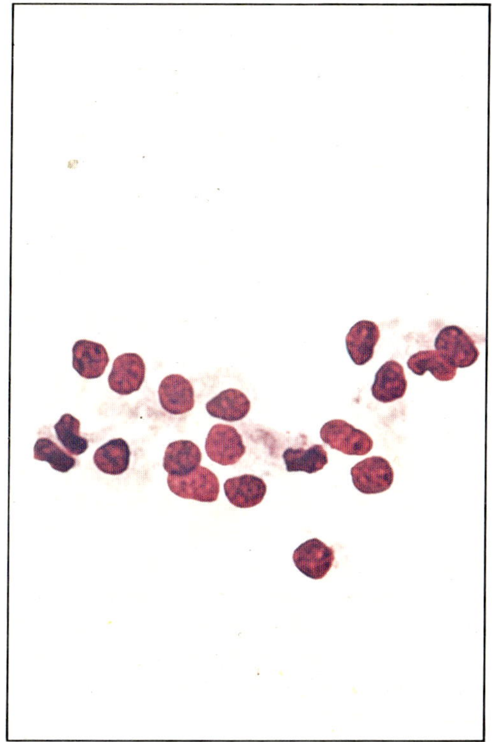

2-11
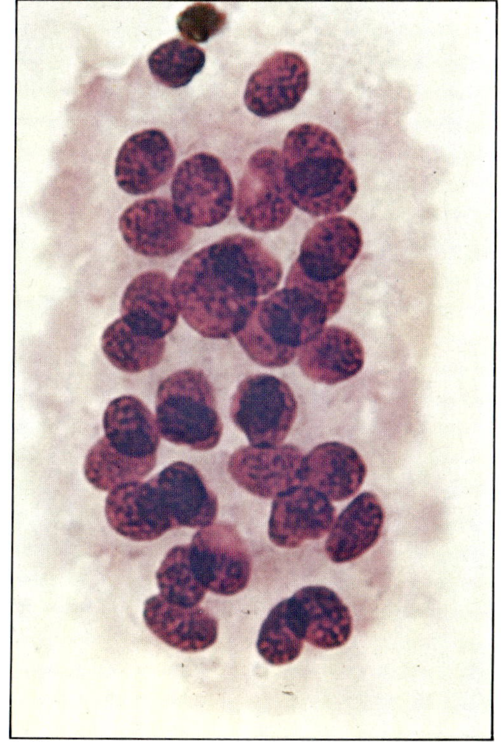

2-12
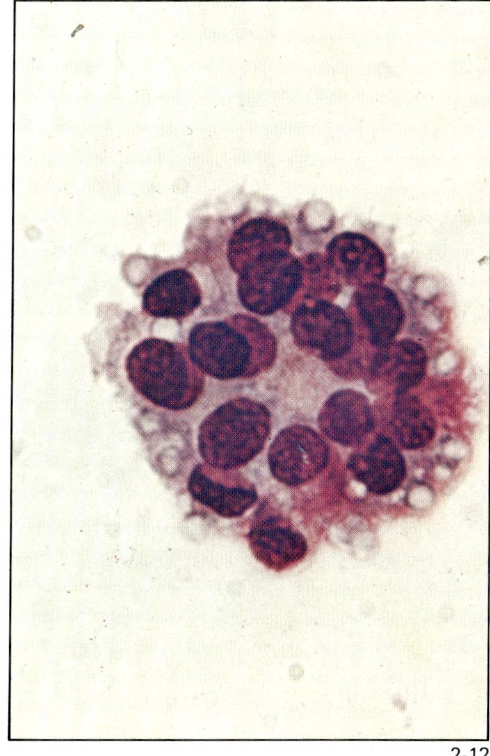

Fig. 2-13 (625×)
Patient L. (control case). Smear preparation of choroid plexus.
The nuclei are round but not hyperchromatic. The cytoplasm may be granulated.

Fig. 2-14 (625×)
Patient L. (control case). Smear preparation of choroid plexus.
There is more crowding of nuclei than in fig. 2-13.

Fig. 2-15 (625×)
Patient T. L.C.S.F. Hydrocephalus. Choroid plexus.
Same characteristics as in the smear preparation.

Fig. 2-16 (625×)
Patient T. L.C.S.F. Hydrocephalus. Choroid plexus.
The nuclei are not hyperchromatic as in ependyma cells
Part of the tissue fragment is free of nuclei.

2-13

2-14

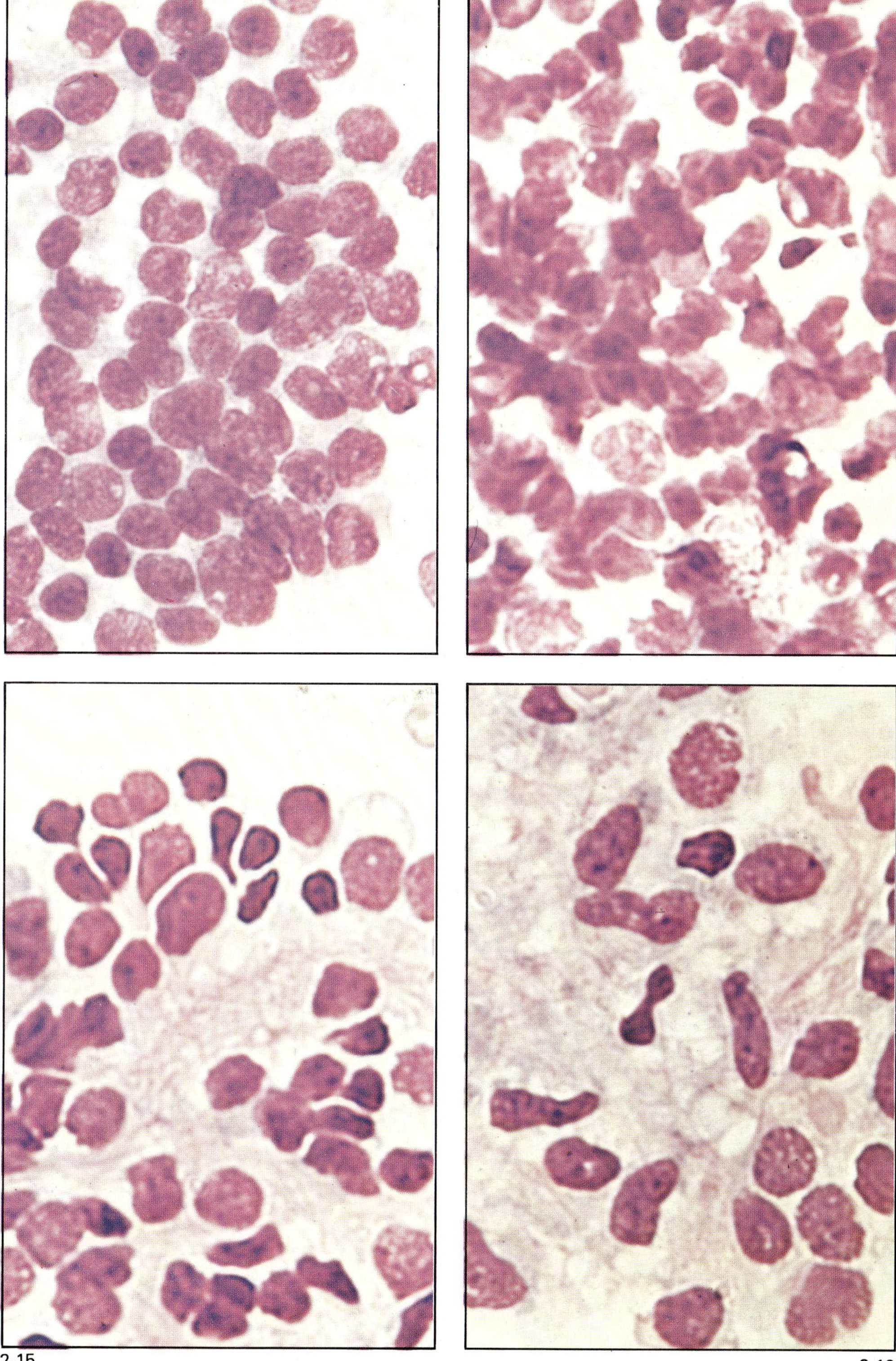

2-15

2-16

Fig. 3-1 (625×)
Patient d.V. Arachnoid hemorrhage. L.C.S.F.
Erythrocytes and a macrophage with two isomorph nuclei.

Fig. 3-2 (625×)
Patient P. Arachnoid hemorrhage. L.C.S.F.
Two macrophages with phagocytosis of black pigment (hemosiderin).

Fig. 3-3 (625×)
Patient d.V. L.C.S.F. Arachnoid hemorrhage.
The arachnoid tissue fragment shows that the so-called histiocytes or
macrophages are in this case activated arachnoid cells phagocytosing
erythrocytes.

Fig. 3-4 (1000×)
Patient R. Hydrocephalus. Spitz-Holter drain. L.C.S.F.
Eosinophil cells can only be diagnosed in a stained preparation and not in a
counting chamber.

Fig. 3-5 (400×)
Patient B. L.C.S.F. Cartilage cells produced by an inexpert lumbar puncture.
They have a burgundy-colored granular cytoplasm, distinct cell borders and dark
red-violet nuclei.

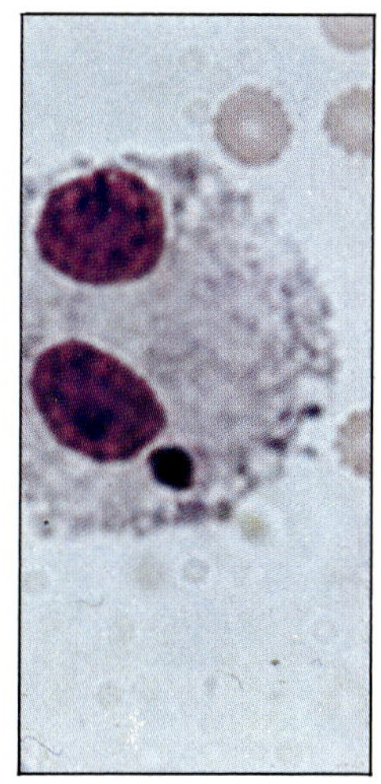

3-1

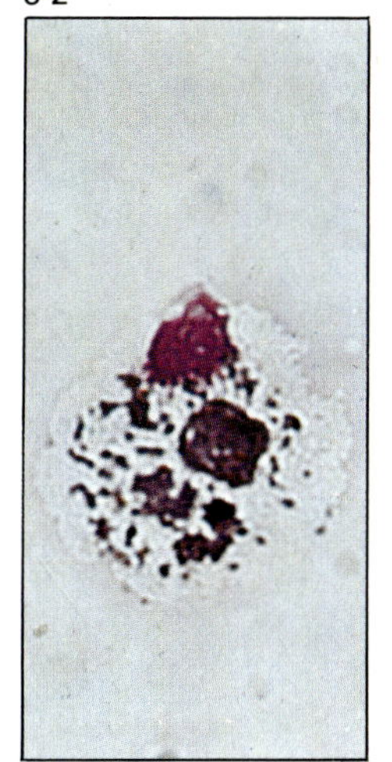

3-2

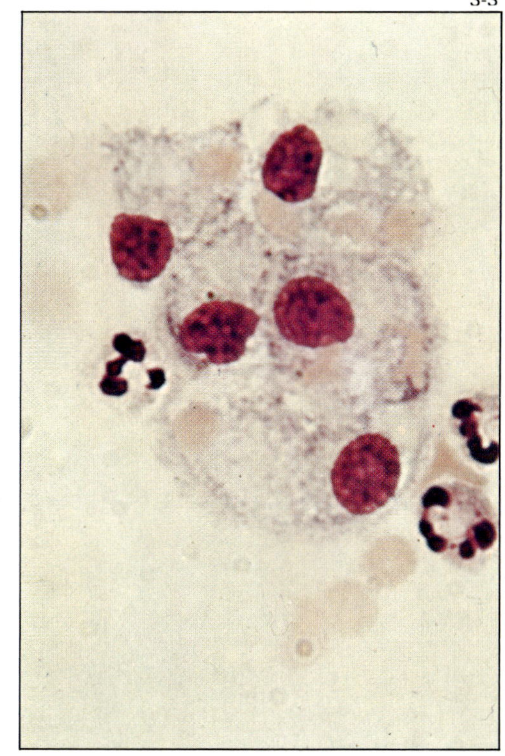

3-3

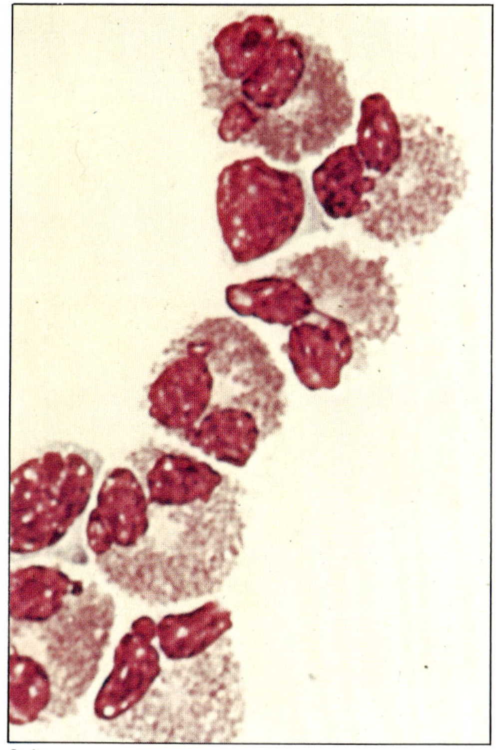

3-4

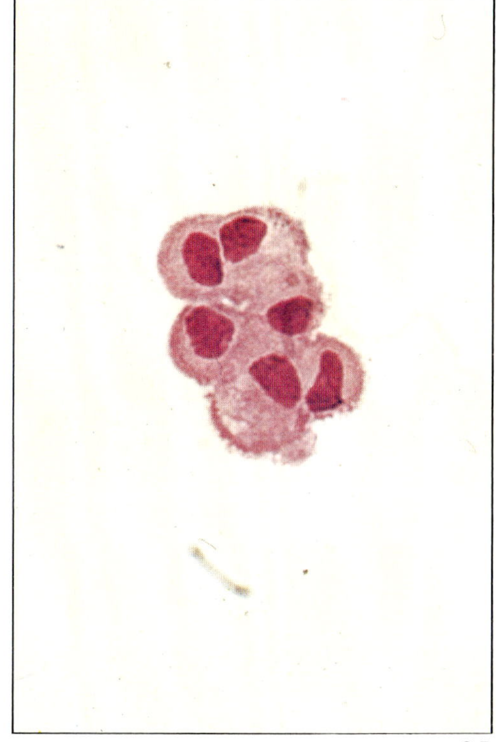

3-5

Fig. 4a-1 (400×)
Patient A. L.C.S.F. Meningitis purulenta. Large numbers of white blood cells.
The majority are neutrophil granulocytes.

Fig. 4a-2 (1000×)
Same patient as in fig. 4a-1. L.C.S.F. Meningitis purulenta.
A large group of extracellular diplococci can be seen in this Jenner–Giemsa
preparation.

Fig. 4a-3 (1000×)
Patient X. Pneumococcal meningitis. Gram staining.
Gram positive extracellular diplococci with capsule.
(Courtesy J.L. Hoogendijk M.D.).

Fig. 4a-4 (1000×)
Patient Y. Meningococcal meningitis. Gram staining.
Gram negative extracellular cocci. The meningococci can be situated intra- and
extracellularly. (Courtesy J.L. Hoogendijk M.D.).

Fig. 4a-5 (1000×)
Patient Z. Cryptococcus meningitis. Gram staining.
The cryptococcus has a capsule and shows 'budding'.
(Courtesy J.L. Hoogendijk M.D.).

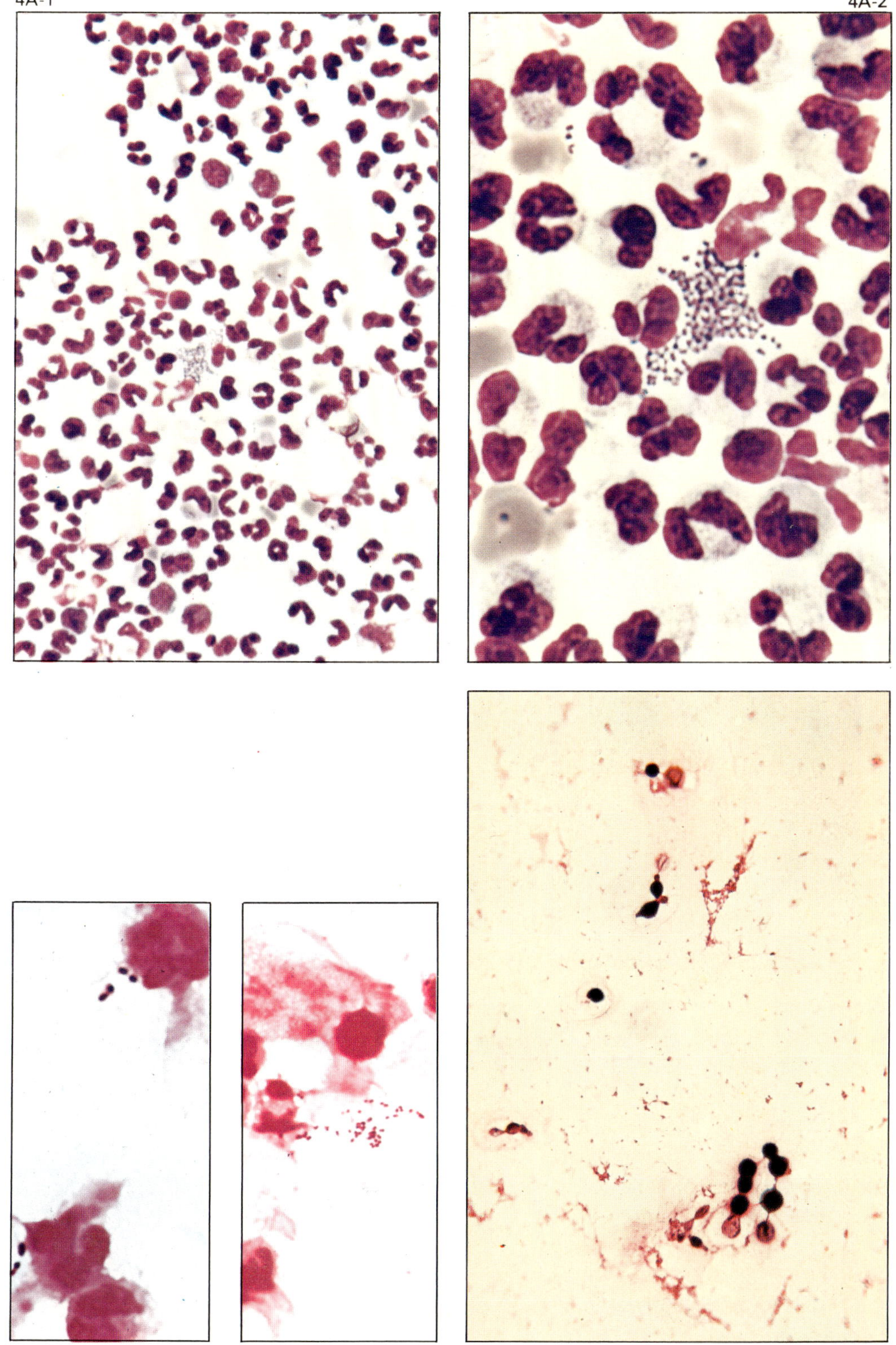
4A-1
4A-2
4A-3
4A-4
4A-5

Fig. 4b-3 (FITC 600 ×)
C.S.F. cells with cytoplasmic fluorescence with pooled anti-ECHO serum.
Note excentric position of nucleus.

Fig. 4b-4 (FITC 600 ×)
C.S.F. cell with cytoplasmic fluorescence with pooled anti-Coxsackie B serum.
Note negative cells.

Fig. 4b-5 (FITC 500 ×)
Polymorphonuclear C.S.F. leukocytes with cytoplasmic fluorescence with a pooled
anti-entero serum.

Fig. 4b-6 (FITC 500 ×)
C.S.F. cells with cytoplasmic fluorescence with anti-polio I serum.
Note polymorphonuclear leukocytes.

4B-3

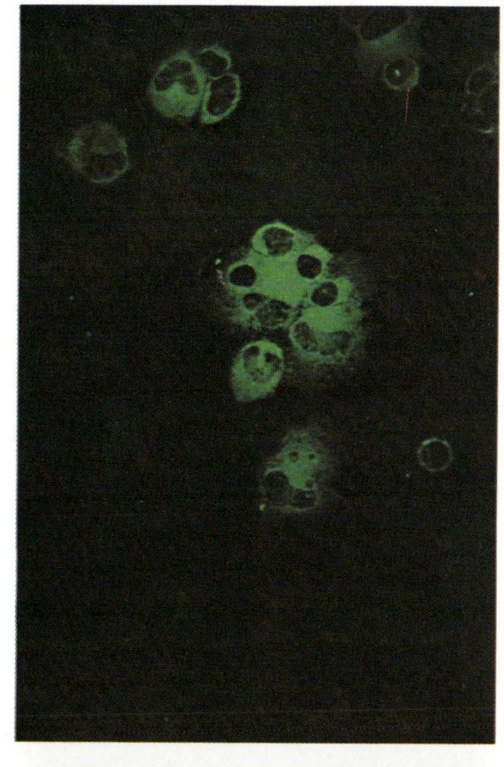

4B-4

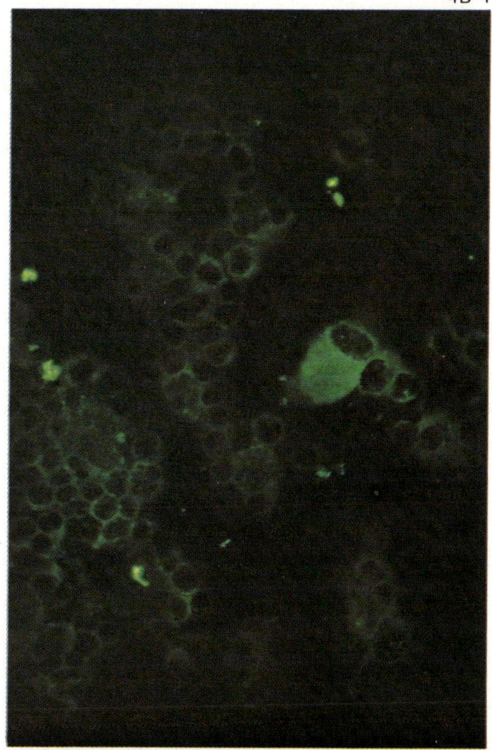

4B-5

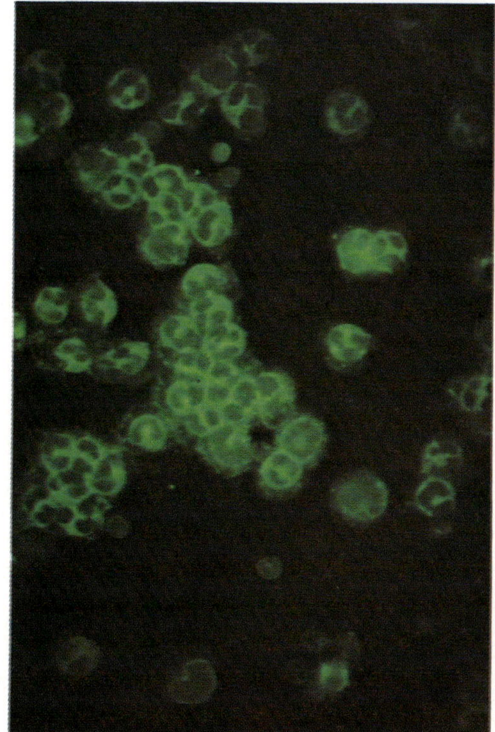

4B-6

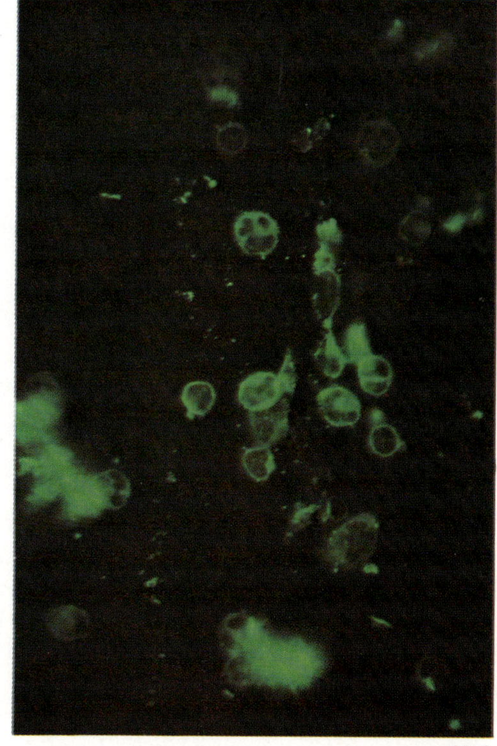

Fig. 4b-7 (FITC 600×)
C.S.F. cell with cytoplasmic fluorescence with anti-mumps serum.
Note negative cells.

Fig. 4b-8 (FITC 400×)
C.S.F. cells with cytoplasmic fluorescence with anti-measles serum in SSPE-case.
Note typical spotted appearance.

Fig. 4b-9 (FITC 320×)
C.S.F. cells with intranuclear fluorescence with anti-simian virus 40 serum.
Note patchy appearance of nucleus.

Fig. 6-1-1 (625×)
Pat.v.d.Zw. L.C.S.F. Left fronto-basal tumor. Astrocytoma grade I.
The cytoplasm is pink. The nuclei show pleomorphism and anisokaryosis.
Nuclear membrane irregularities.

Fig. 6-1-2 (625×)
Same patient as in fig. 6-1-1. L.C.S.F. Left fronto-basal tumor.
Astrocytoma grade I. The nuclei have irregular contours.

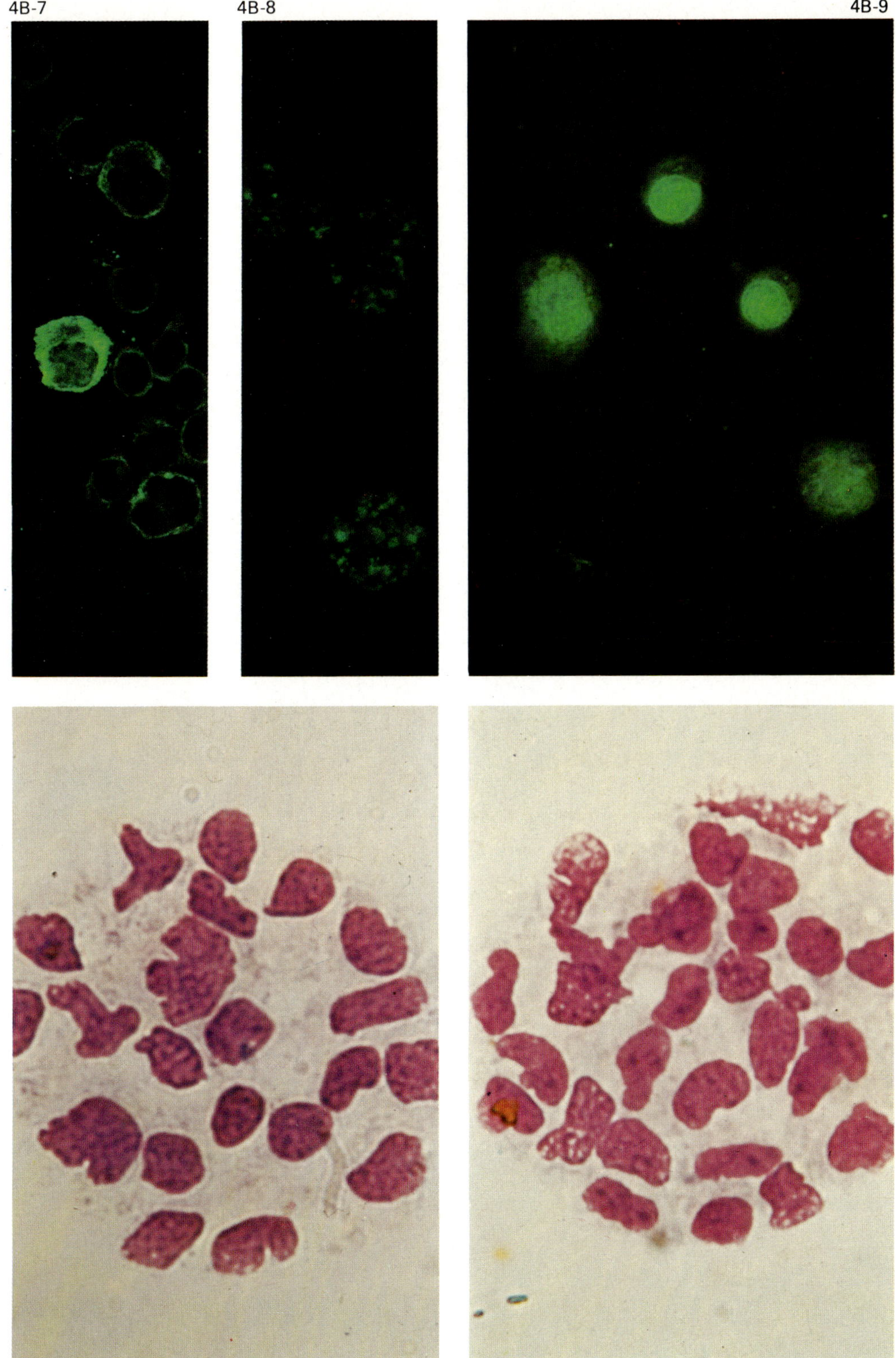

4B-7
4B-8
4B-9
6-1-1
6-1-2

Fig. 6-1-3 (625×)
Same patient as in fig. 6-1-1. L.C.S.F. Left fronto-basal tumor.
Astrocytoma grade I. Chromatin clumping of the nuclei and irregular contours.

Fig. 6-1-4 (625×)
Same patient as in fig. 6-1-1. L.C.S.F. Left fronto-basal tumor.
Astrocytoma grade I. Here, the cytoplasm is mauve colored and the nuclei are
more polymorph.

Fig. 6-1-5 (625×)
Patient S.V. V.C.S.F. Brain stem tumor at autopsy. Astrocytoma grade I-II.
There is not much polymorphism.

Fig. 6-1-6 (625×)
Patient S.V. V.C.S.F. Brain stem tumor at autopsy. Astrocytoma grade I-II.
There is some anisokaryosis and nuclear hyperchromasia.

6-1-3

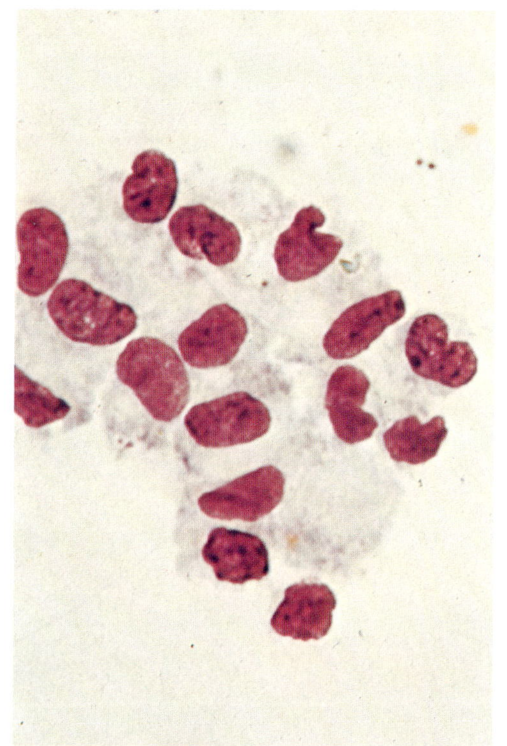

6-1-4

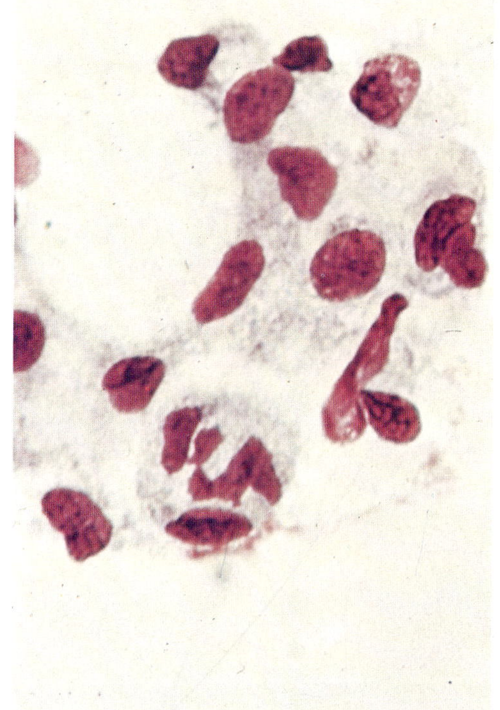

6-1-5

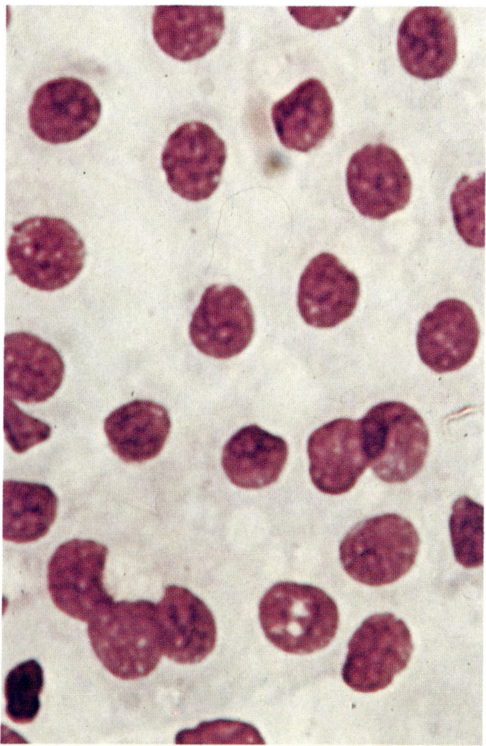

6-1-6

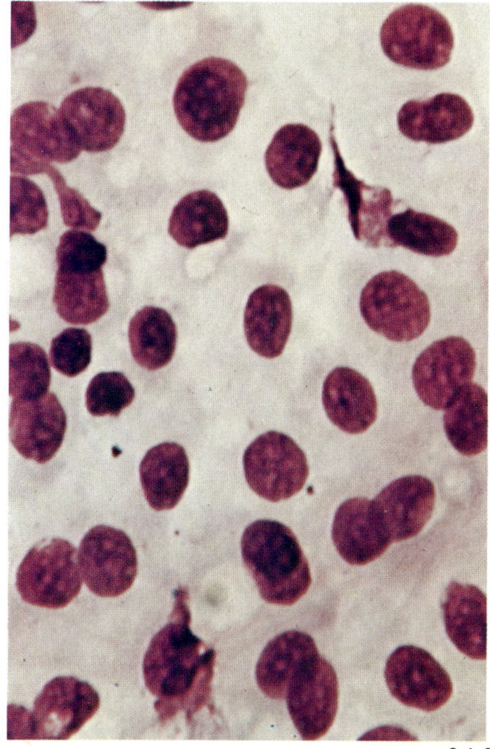

Fig. 6-1-7 (625×)
Patient v.d.B. L.C.S.F. Thalamic tumor at autopsy. Astrocytoma grade I-II.
There is no crowding but variation in size and shape of the nuclei.

Fig. 6-1-8 (625×)
Patient v.d.B. L.C.S.F. Thalamic tumor at autopsy. Astrocytoma grade I-II.
A tissue sheet which in itself is not proving a tumor.
However, it was of the same preparation as that of fig. 6-1-7.

Fig. 6-1-9 (400×)
Patient B.Z. Cyst aspirate. Left parietal tumor. Astrocytoma grade I-II.
Resemblance of the tumor cells in this cyst aspirate with those in the spinal fluid
of astrocytoma grade I and I-II. Slight anisokaryosis. Prominent nucleoli.
Cells sometimes rounded, sometimes bipolar. Cytoplasm light blue.

Fig. 6-1-10 (625×)
Patient St. V.C.S.F. Left temporal tumor. Astrocytoma grade II.
A tissue fragment with crowded nuclei. There is anisokaryosis and chromatin
clumping. The cytoplasm is mauve colored.

6-1-7

6-1-8

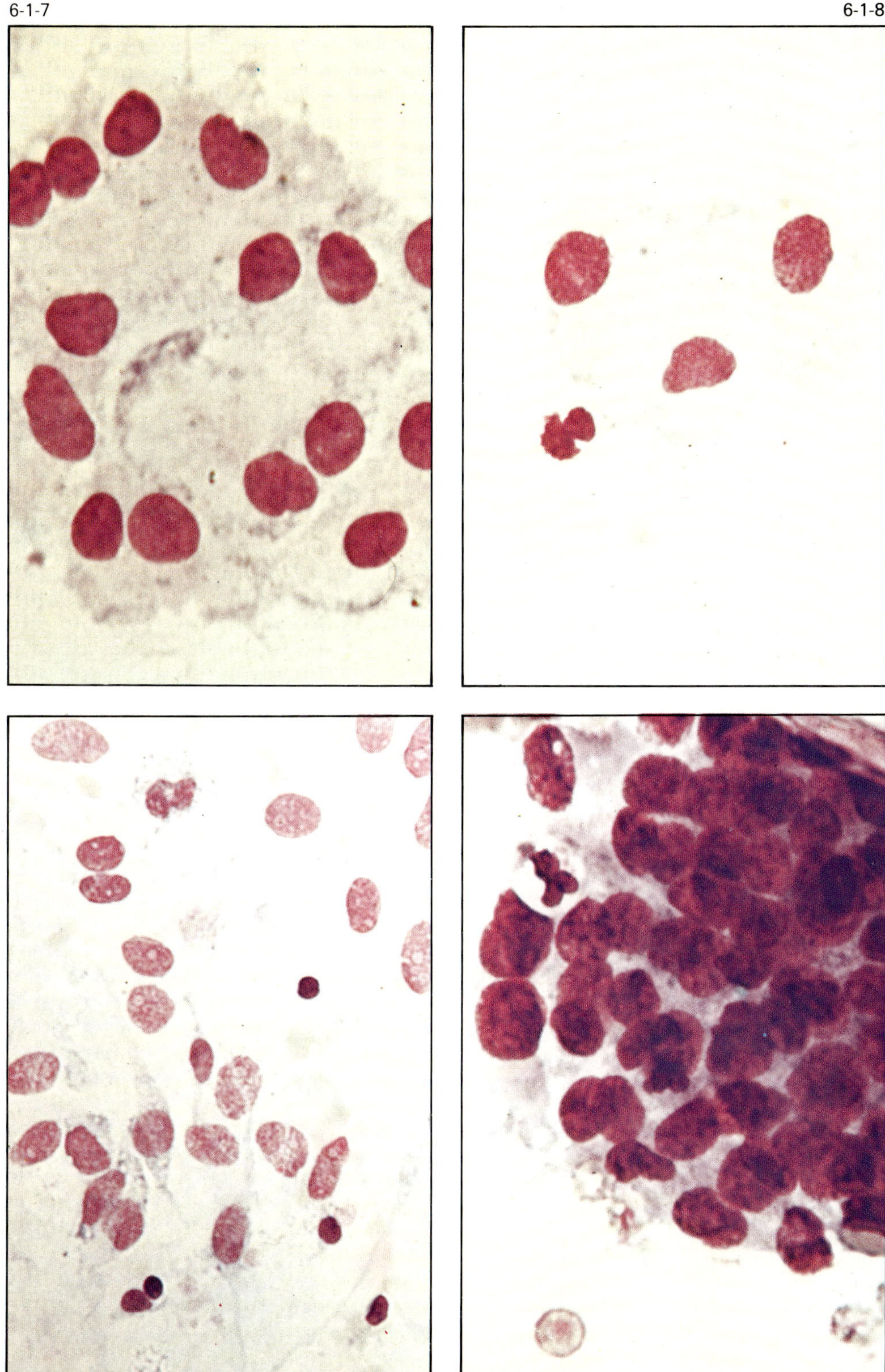

6-1-9

6-1-10

Fig. 6-1-11 (625×)
Same patient as in fig. 6-1-10. V.C.S.F. Left temporal tumor.
Astrocytoma grade II. Less crowding of nuclei.
There is more cytoplasm visible.

Fig. 6-1-12 (625×)
Same patient as in fig. 6-1-10. V.C.S.F. Left temporal tumor.
Astrocytoma grade II. There is more polymorphism of the nuclei than in
fig. 6-1-10 and 6-1-11. The nuclei are hyperchromatic.

Fig. 6-1-13 (625×)
Same patient as in fig. 6-1-10. V.C.S.F. Left temporal tumor.
Astrocytoma grade II. Slight vacuolisation of the nuclei possibly caused by
autolysis.

Fig. 6-1-14 (625×)
Patient Si. V.C.S.F. Right fronto-parietal-temporal tumor.
Astrocytoma grade II-III. A sheet of tumor cells with pink and light blue
cytoplasm. There is anisokaryosis, chromatin clumping and pleomorphism of the
nuclei.

6-1-11

6-1-12

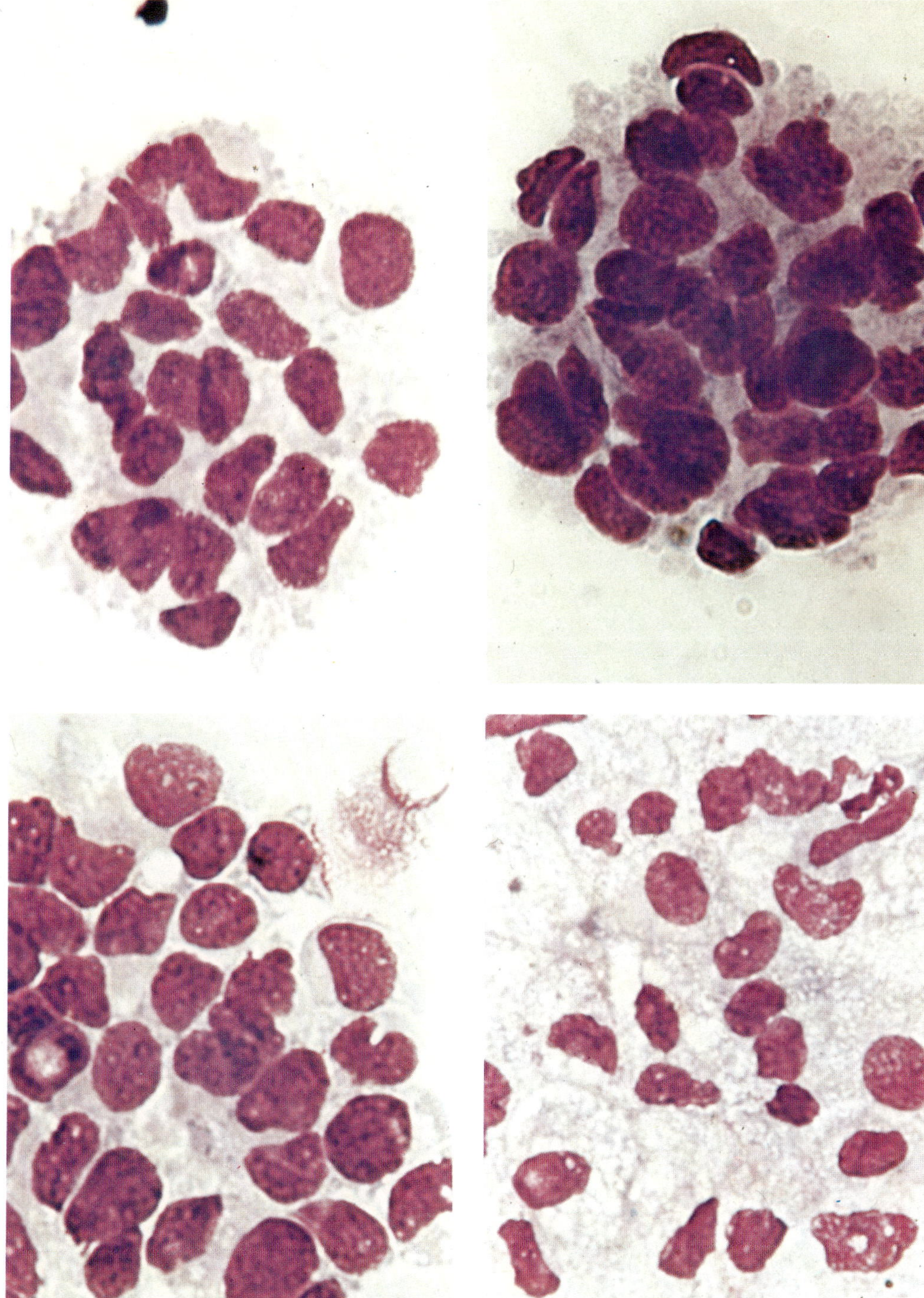

6-1-13

6-1-14

Fig. 6-1-15 (625×)
Same patient as in fig. 6-1-14. V.C.S.F. Right fronto-parietal-temporal tumor.
Astrocytoma grade II-III. The cytoplasm is basophil.
A sheet of tumor cells in which one cell is far too large and has four nuclei (giant
tumor cell).

Fig. 6-1-16 (625×)
Same patient as in fig. 6-1-14. V.C.S.F. Right fronto-parietal-temporal tumor.
Astrocytoma grade II-III. The cell borders are well defined.

Fig. 6-1-17 (625×)
Same patient as in fig. 6-1-14. V.C.S.F. Right fronto-parietal-temporal tumor.
Astrocytoma grade II-III. Giant tumor cell with four nuclei next to a small tumor
cell with a large nucleus.

Fig. 6-1-18 (625×)
Patient Sch. V.C.S.F. Cerebellar tumor. Astrocytoma grade III.
A tissue sheet with crowded nuclei.
There is anisokaryosis, pleomorphism and chromatin clumping.
The cytoplasm is mauve colored.

6-1-15

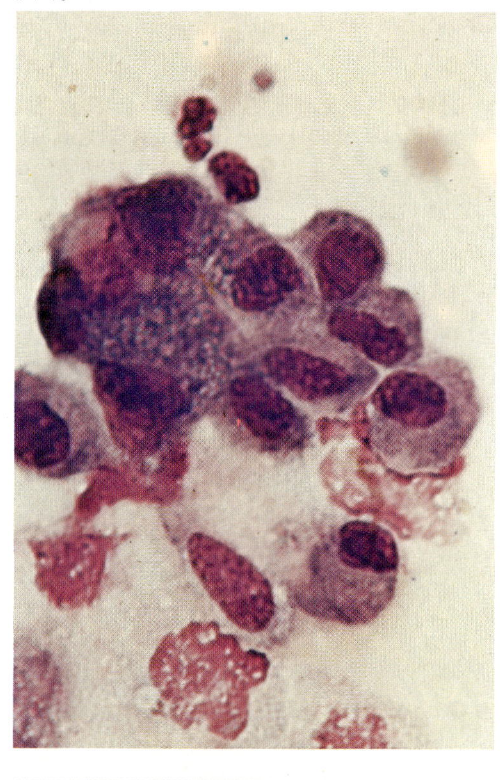

6-1-16

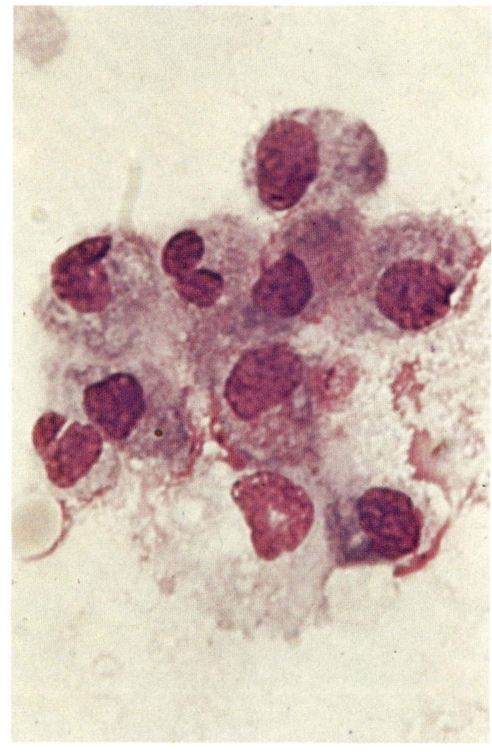

6-1-17

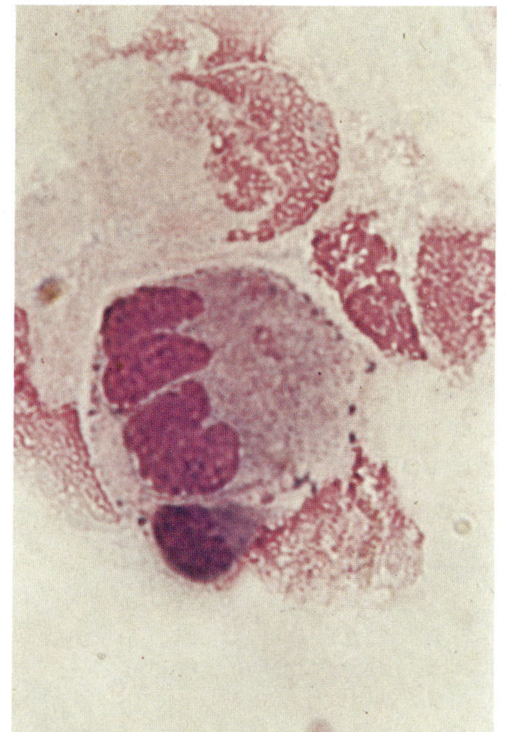

6-1-18

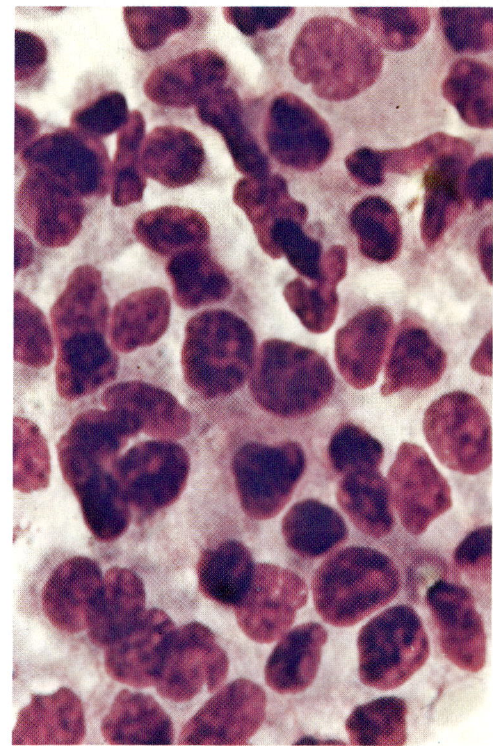

Fig. 6-1-19 (625 ×)
Same patient as in fig. 6-1-18. V.C.S.F. Cerebellar tumor.
Astrocytoma grade III. Bizarre formed nuclei.

Fig. 6-1-20 (625 ×)
Patient M. V.C.S.F. Corpus callosum tumor. Astrocytoma grade III.
This was the only sheet of tumor cells in this C.S.F. preparation.
Marked polymorphism. The nucleus–cytoplasm ratio is strongly in favor of the
nuclei. This preparation could be easily misdiagnosed as medulloblastoma.

Fig. 6-1-21 (625 ×)
Patient T. V.C.S.F. Cerebellar tumor. Astrocytoma grade III.
Mauve colored cytoplasm. Strong polymorphism. Distinct cell contours.

Fig. 6-1-22 (400 ×)
Patient v.W. Cyst aspirate. Left parieto-occipital tumor. Astrocytoma grade III.
A sheet of tumor cells with a relatively minor anisokaryosis.
The cytoplasm is light blue and vacuolated by autolysis.

6-1-19

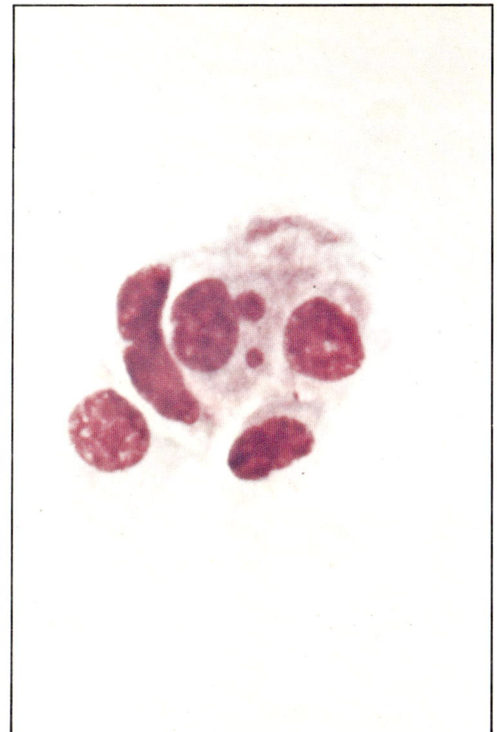

6-1-20

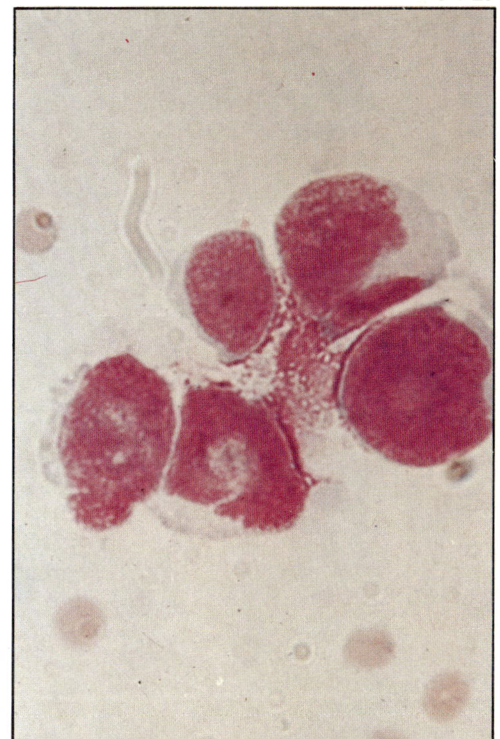

6-1-21

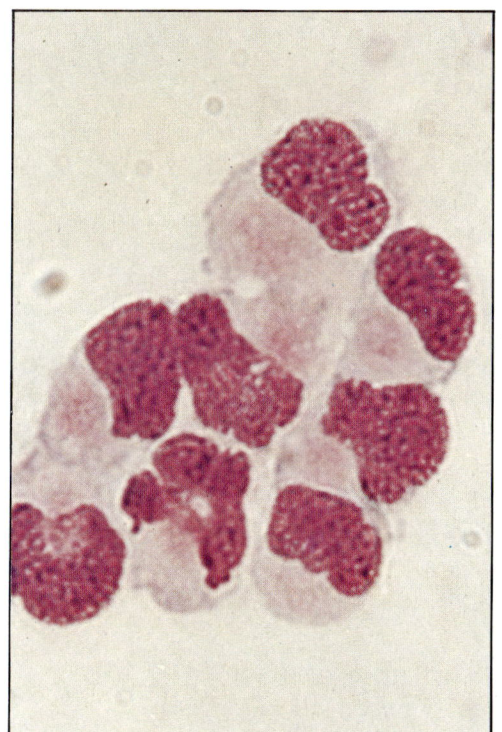

6-1-22

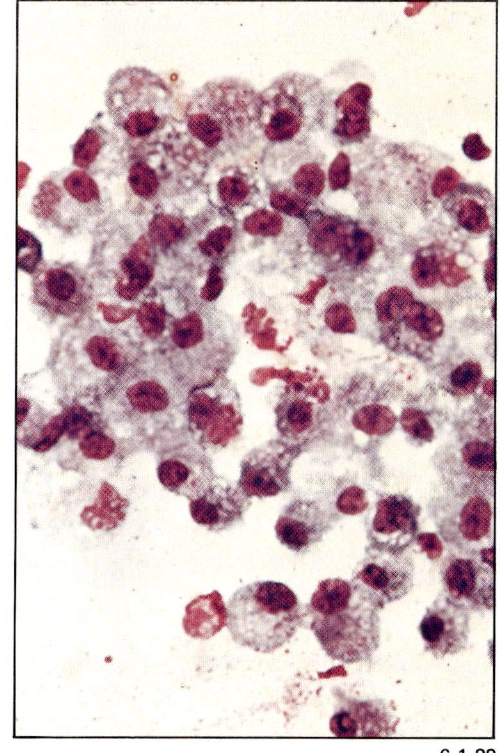

Fig. 6-1-23 (400×)
Patient Sch. Cyst aspirate. Astrocytoma grade III.
A sheet of tumor cells with marked anisokaryosis and anisocytosis.
The morphology differs much from, for example, fig. 6-1-22.

Fig. 6-1-24 (625×)
Patient Z.V.D. S.C.S.F. Right frontal tumor. Astrocytoma grade III-IV.
A sheet of tumor cells with very large and bizarre nuclei, prominent nucleoli and
mitosis (telophase). The cytoplasm is mauve colored and the cell borders have a
sharp outline.

Fig. 6-1-25 (625×)
Same patient as in fig. 6-1-24. S.C.S.F. Astrocytoma grade III-IV.
Clover leaf nuclei with prominent nucleoli.

Fig. 6-1-26 (400×)
Same patient as in fig. 6-1-24. S.C.S.F. Astrocytoma grade III-IV.
Marked polymorphism of the nuclei. More pronounced hyperchromasia. There is
phagocytosis of bloodpigment.

6-1-23

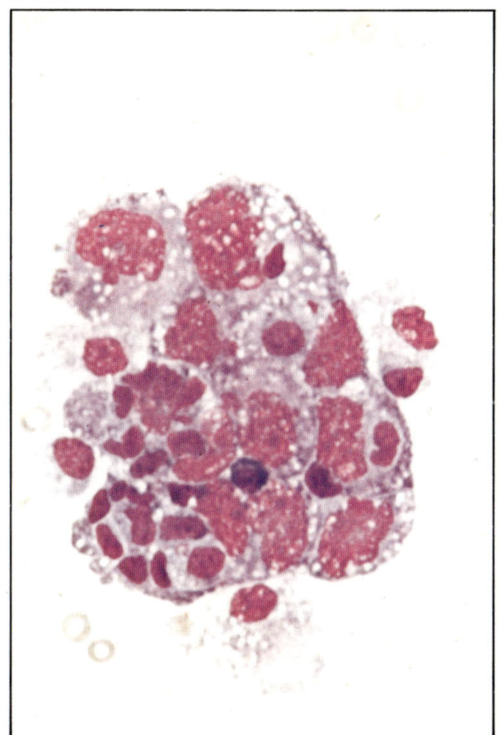

6-1-24

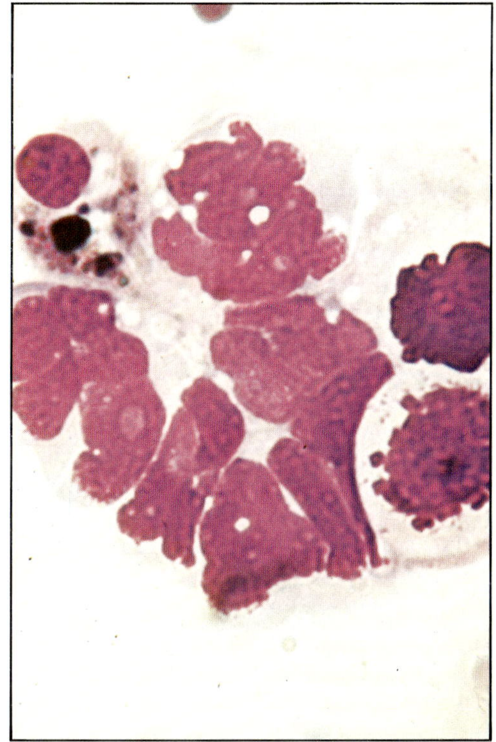

6-1-25

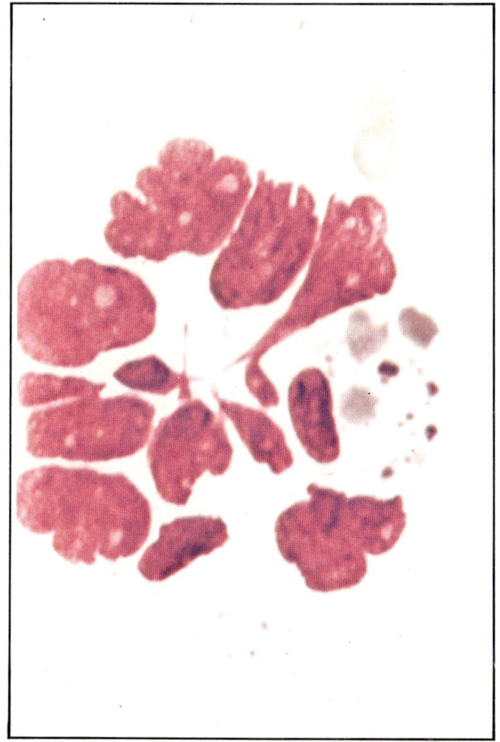

6-1-26

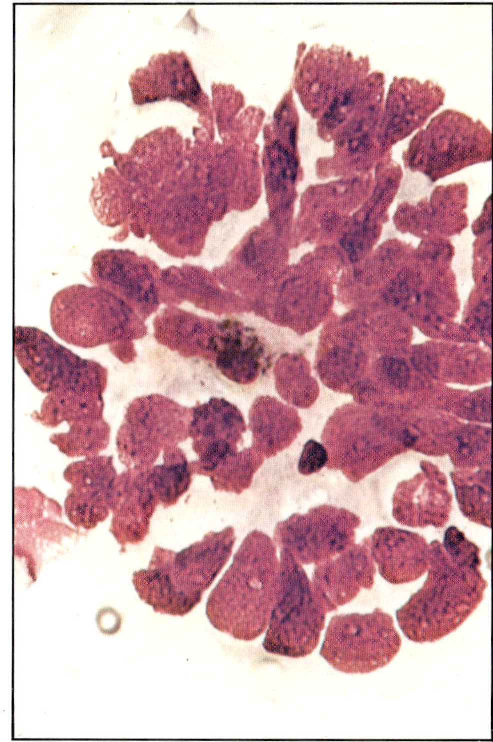

Fig. 6-1-27 (400×)
Same patient as in fig. 6-1-24. S.C.S.F. Astrocytoma grade III-IV.
Pronounced anisokaryosis and hyperchromasia. There is also phagocytosis of
blood pigment. Crowding and pleomorphism of the nuclei.

Fig. 6-1-28 (625×)
Patient v.D. L.C.S.F. Right temporal tumor. Astrocytoma grade IV (glioblastoma
multiforme). Light blue colored cytoplasm.
Pronounced anisokaryosis and distinct cell borders.

Fig. 6-1-29 (625×)
Same patient as in fig. 6-1-28. L.C.S.F. Right temporal tumor. Astrocytoma grade IV.
Very marked anisokaryosis, crowding and pleomorphism of the nuclei.

Fig. 6-1-30 (625×)
Same patient as in fig. 6-1-28. L.C.S.F. Right temporal tumor. Astrocytoma grade IV.
Marked anisokaryosis and nuclear polymorphism.

6-1-27

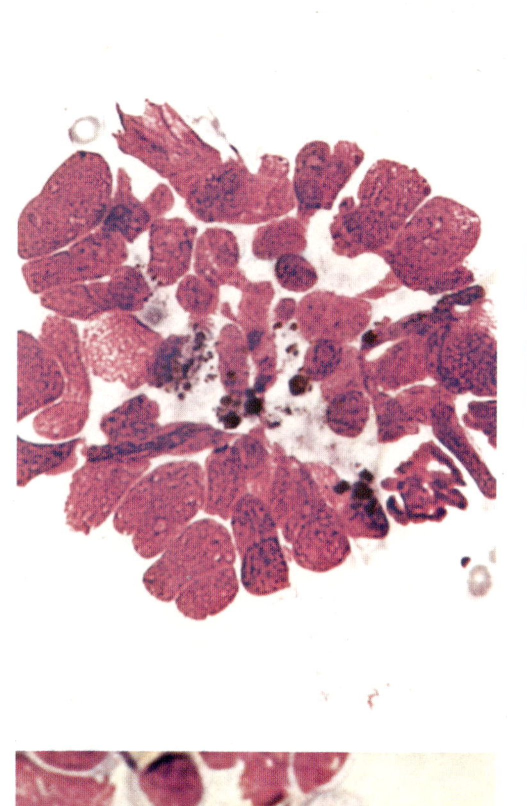

6-1-28

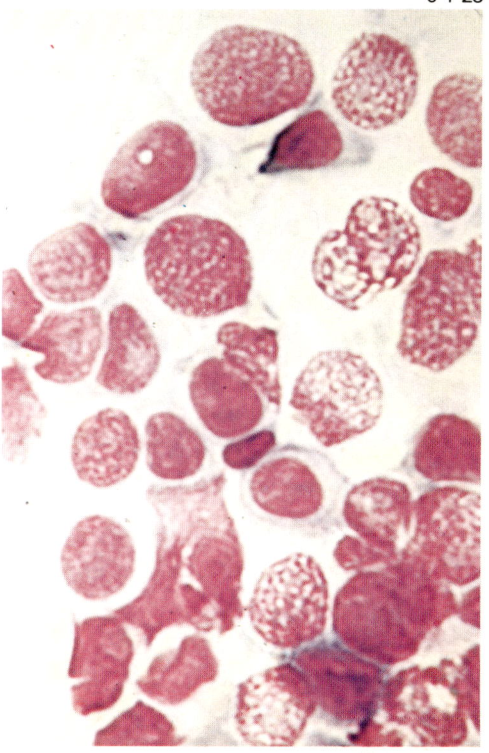

6-1-29

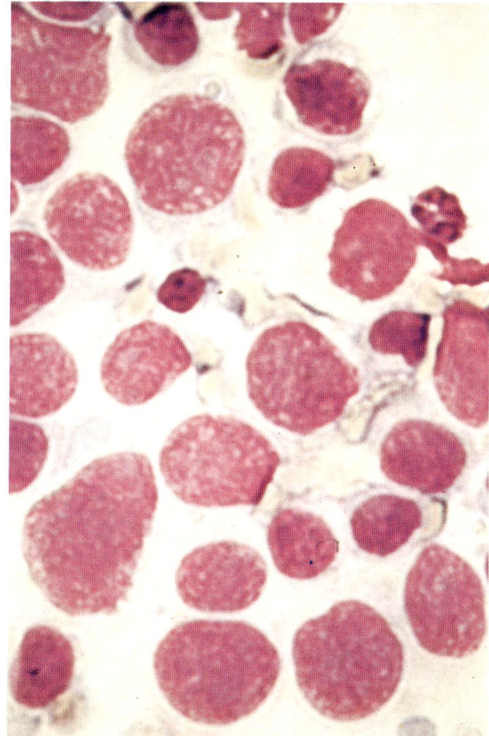

6-1-30

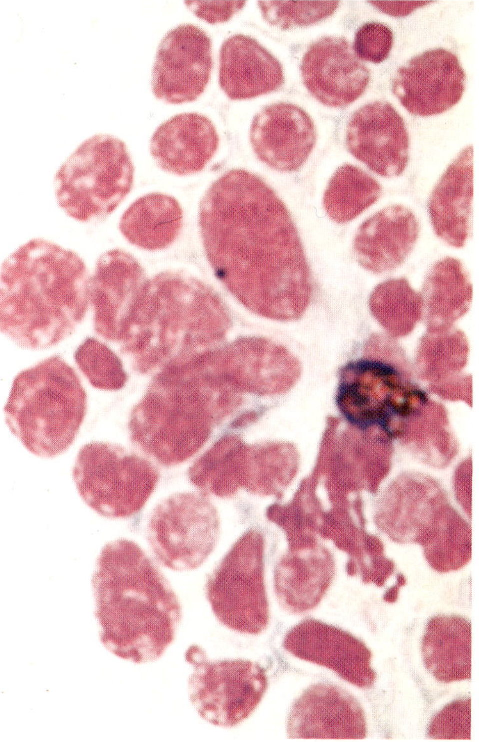

Fig. 6-1-31 (400×)
Same patient as in fig. 6-1-28. L.C.S.F. Right temporal tumor. Astrocytoma grade IV.
Free lying tumor cells. The anisocytosis is more evident than in tissue sheets.
Furthermore, one cell with two nuclei of different shape.

Fig. 6-1-32 (625×)
Same patient as in fig. 6-1-28. L.C.S.F. Right temporal tumor. Astrocytoma grade IV.
Giant tumor cell. The cytoplasm is blue—violet.
The nuclei are of different size.

Fig. 6-1-33 (625×)
Same patient as in fig. 6-1-28. L.C.S.F. Right temporal tumor. Astrocytoma grade IV.
Giant tumor cell with abnormal mitosis. The cytoplasm is light blue.

Fig. 6-1-34 (625×)
Same patient as in 6-1-28. L.C.S.F. Right temporal tumor. Astrocytoma grade IV.
Free lying tumor cells. Anisokaryosis. The cytoplasm is mauve colored.
One cell is in mitosis.

6-1-31

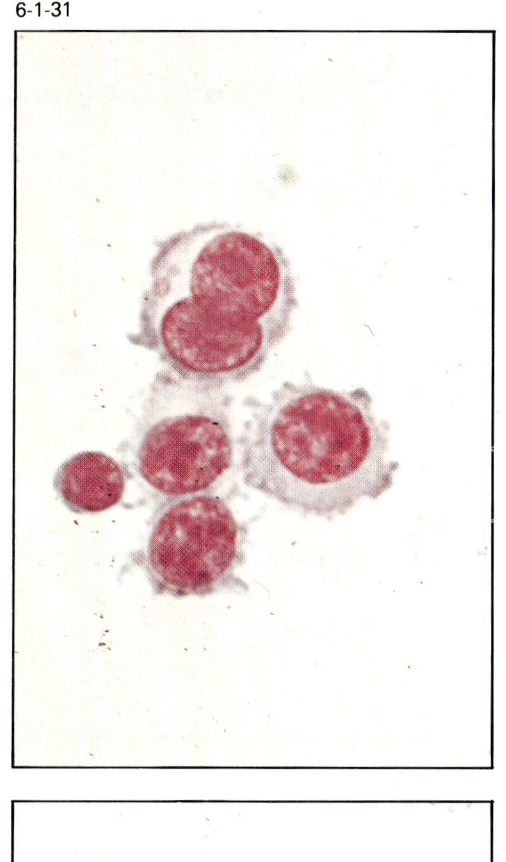

6-1-32

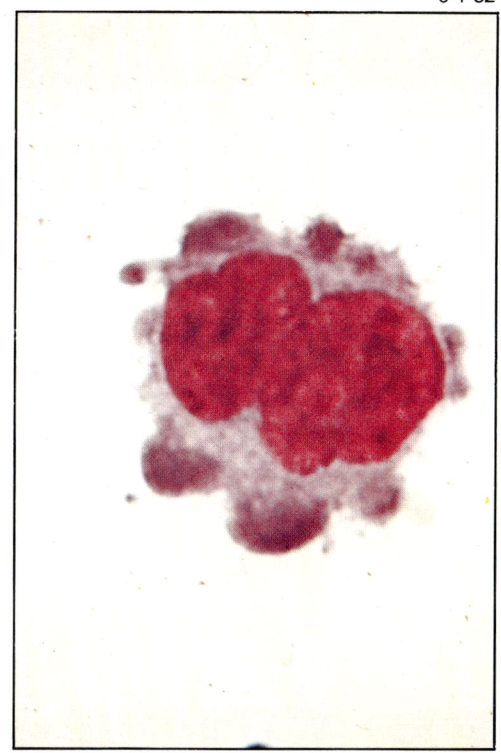

6-1-33

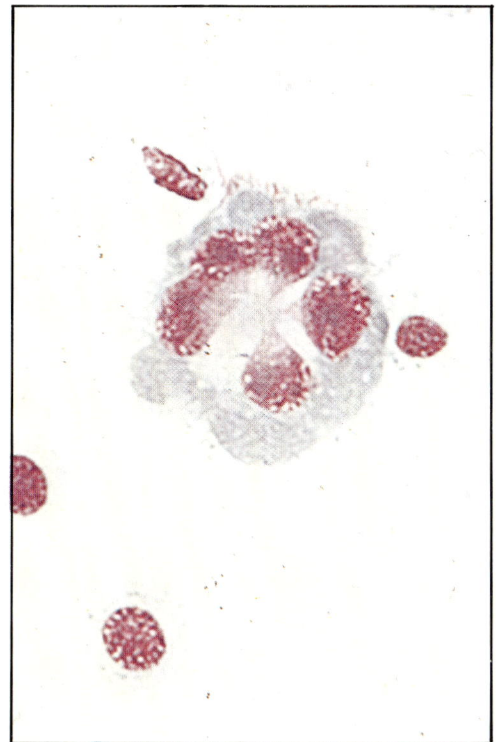

6-1-34

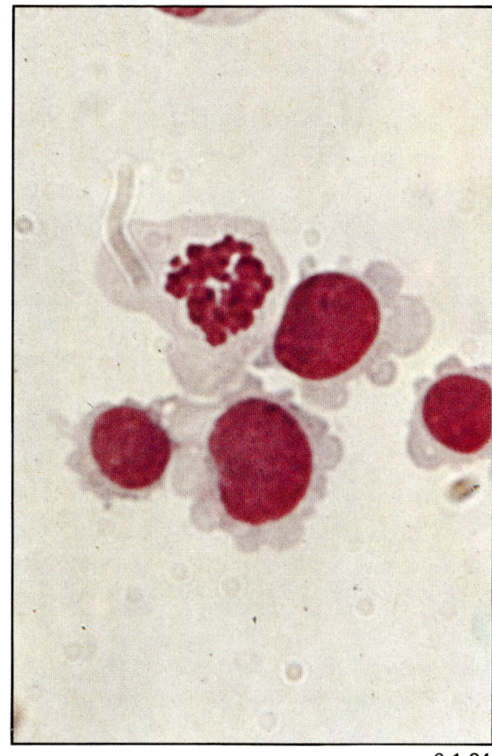

Fig. 6-2-1 (400×)
Patient B. L.C.S.F. Medulloblastoma + transverse lesion.
The sheet of tumor cells shows anisocytosis and anisokaryosis.
The cytoplasm is violet. There is ganglionic differentiation.

Fig. 6-2-2 (625×)
Same case as in fig. 6-2-1. L.C.S.F. Medulloblastoma. Typical picture.
There is crowding of nuclei. The nucleus-cytoplasm ratio is very high.
Very pronounced pleomorphism.

Fig. 6-2-3 (400×)
Same case as in fig. 6-2-1. L.C.S.F. Medulloblastoma.
This tissue fragment has the same characteristics as that in fig. 6-2-1.
This picture is not typical for a medulloblastoma.
There is pronounced ganglionic differentiation.

Fig. 6-2-4 (625×)
Same case as in fig. 6-2-1. L.C.S.F. Typical picture of a medulloblastoma.
Same characteristics as fig. 6-2-2.

6-2-1

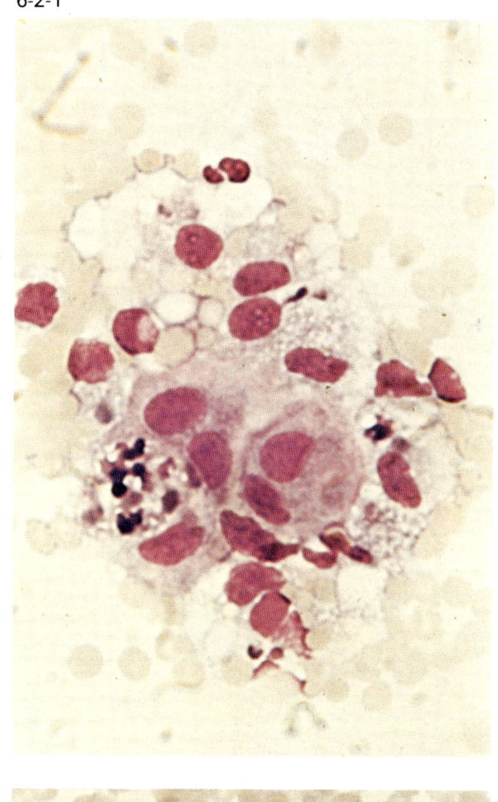

6-2-2

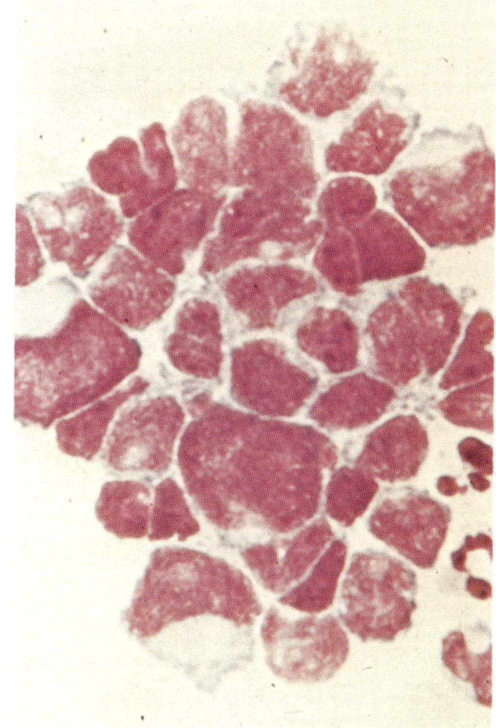

6-2-3

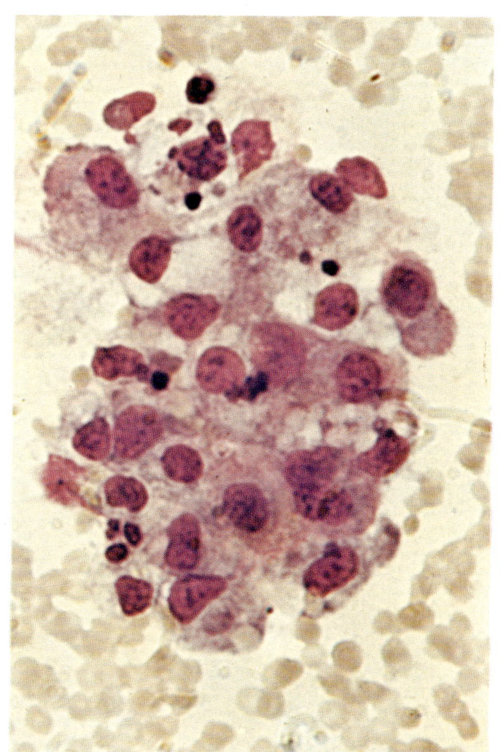

6-2-4

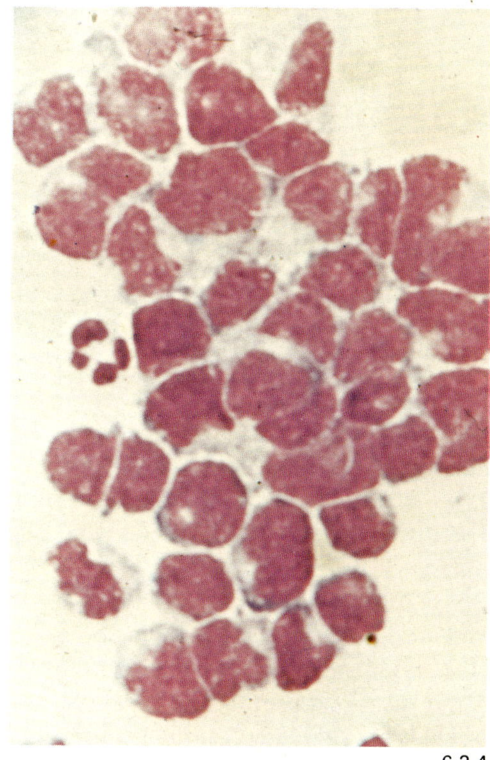

Fig. 6-2-5 (400 ×)
Same case as in fig. 6-2-1. L.C.S.F. Medulloblastoma.
Pronounced crowding of nuclei. A specific diagnosis is not possible.

Fig. 6-2-6 (625 ×)
Same case as in fig. 6-2-1. L.C.S.F. Medulloblastoma.
Tissue fragment of medulloblastoma. Differentiation with retinoblastoma is
difficult.

Fig. 6-2-7 (625 ×)
Patient L. L.C.S.F. Medulloblastoma. Another type of this polymorph tumor.
There are many small nucleoli, crowding and pleomorphism of nuclei.
The nucleus – cytoplasm ratio is very high.

Fig. 6-2-8 (250 ×)
Patient B. L.C.S.F. Medulloblastoma.
Two tissue sheets of medulloblastoma tumor cells.
A mitosis is present in one of the tissue sheets.
Mitoses are regularly found in tumor fragments. Overview 250 × .

6-2-5
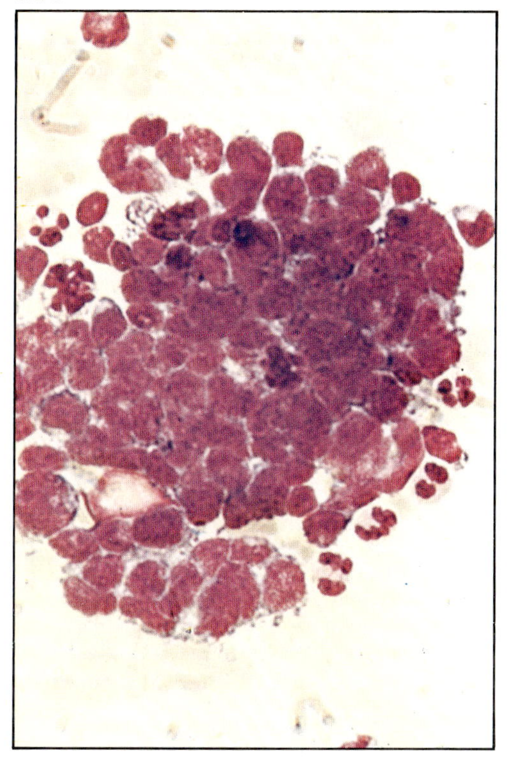

6-2-6
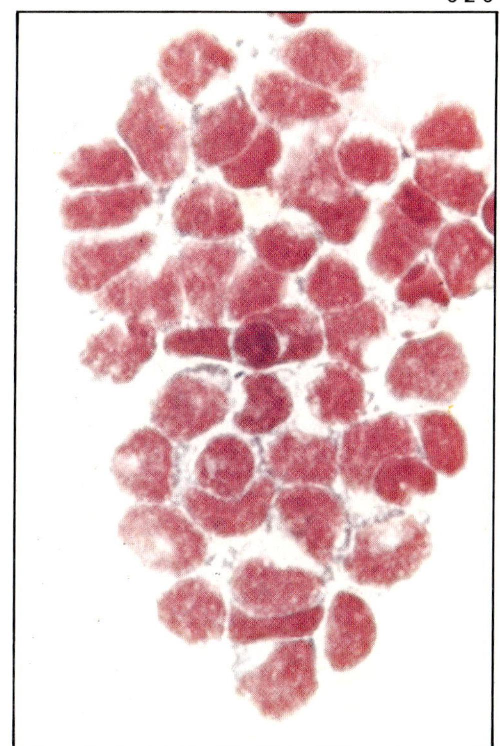

6-2-7
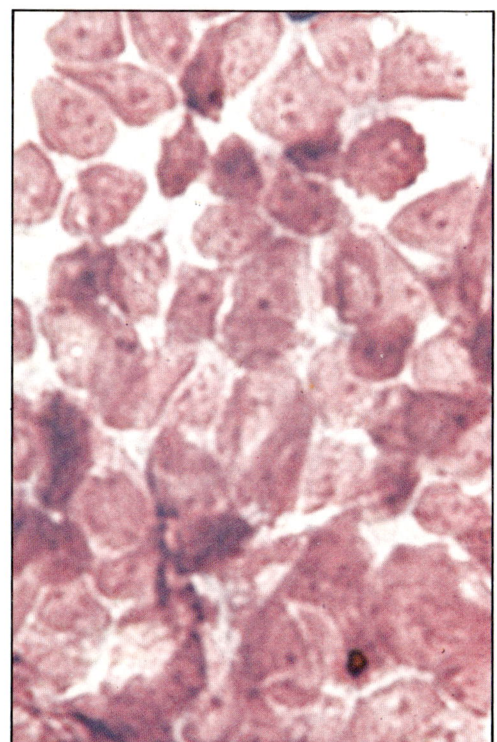

6-2-8
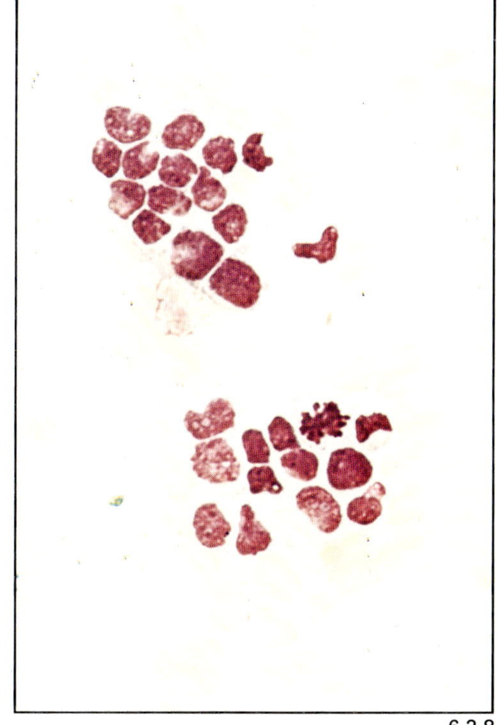

Fig. 6-3-1 (625 ×)
Patient Z. V.C.S.F. Cerebellar tumor. Ependymoma.
A tissue fragment of tumor cells with light-violet cytoplasm.
The nuclei are crowded and hyperchromatic.
Marked resemblance with ependyma in C.S.F. (see figs. 2-11 and 2-12).

Fig. 6-3-2 (400 ×)
Patient Z. V.C.S.F. Cerebellar tumor. Ependymoma.
A sheet of tumor cells with rosette formation.
The nuclei show a pronounced variation in size and shape.

Fig. 6-3-3 (625 ×)
Patient Z. V.C.S.F. Cerebellar tumor. Ependymoma.
A tissue fragment of tumor cells with a giant nucleus.
Typical reticulated structure of the chromatin in the nuclei.

Fig. 6-3-4 (625 ×)
Patient Z. V.C.S.F. Cerebellar tumor. Ependymoma.
A sheet of tumor cells with marked anisokaryosis and hyperchromasia.

71

6-3-1
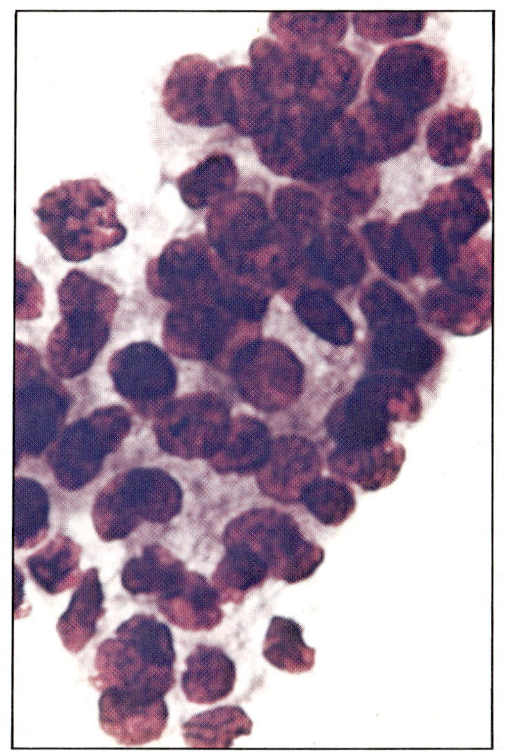

6-3-2
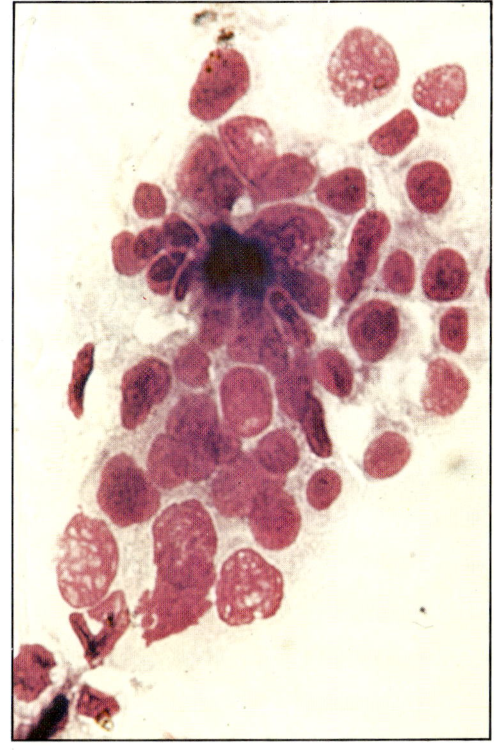

6-3-3
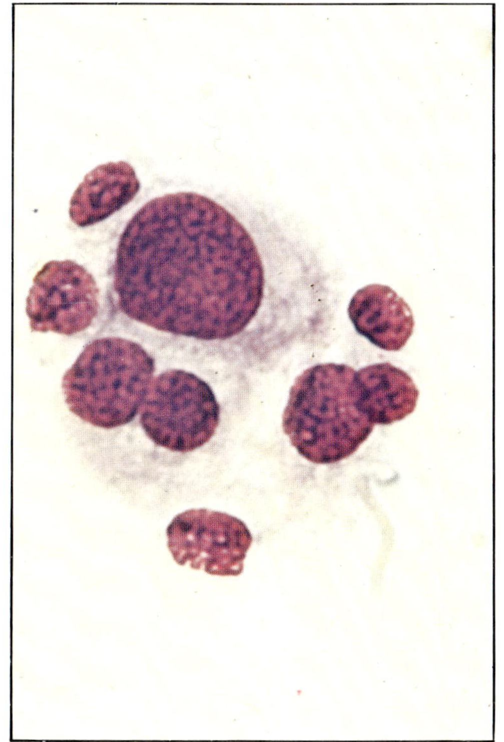

6-3-4
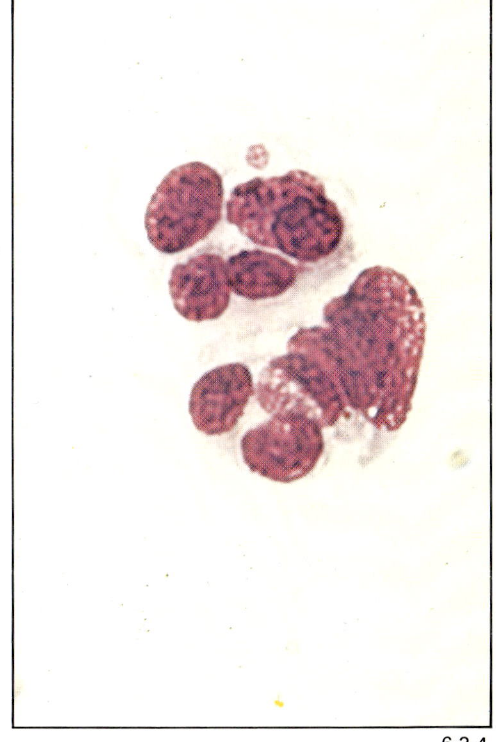

Fig. 6-3-5 (625 ×)
Patient Z. V.C.S.F. Cerebellar tumor. Ependymoma.
A large tissue fragment of tumor cells with the typical characteristics of
ependyma but with an evident variation of size and shape of the nuclei.

Fig. 6-3-6 (625 ×)
Patient Z. V.C.S.F. Cerebellar tumor. Ependymoma.
An other example of a sheet of tumor cells.

Fig. 6-3-7 (625 ×)
Patient Z. V.C.S.F. Cerebellar tumor. Ependymoma.
The nuclei in this tissue sheet are not very polymorph.
However, one nucleus is in mitosis.

Fig. 6-3-8 (625 ×)
Patient Z. Cerebellar tumor. Ependymoma.
Routine paraffin hematoxylin-eosin preparation.
Rosette formation and a mitosis.
Note the large difference in morphology between C.S.F. cell preparation and
paraffin sections.

6-3-5
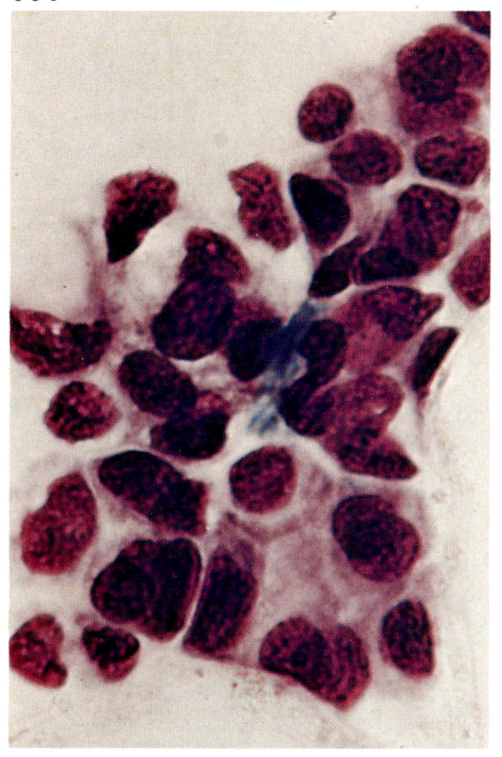

6-3-6
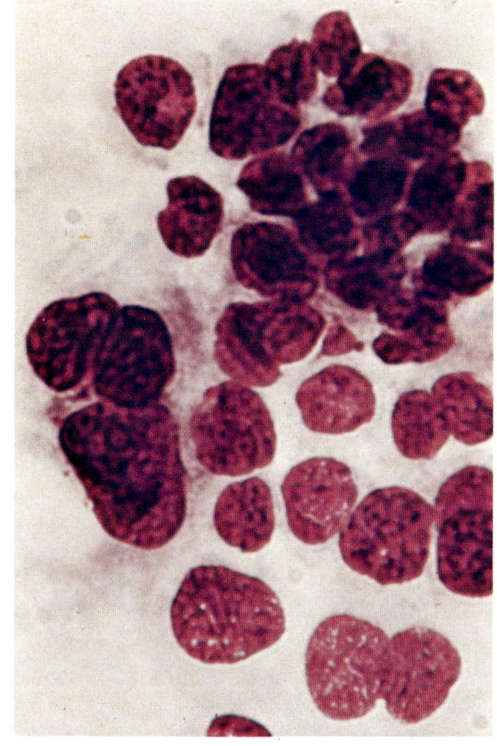

6-3-7
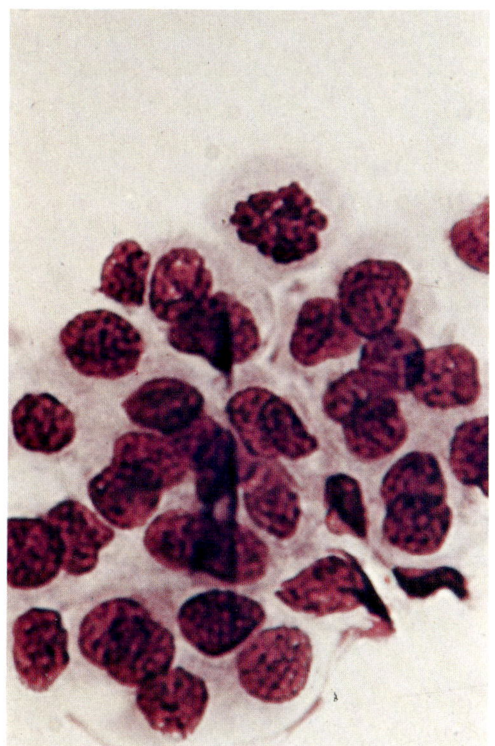

6-3-8
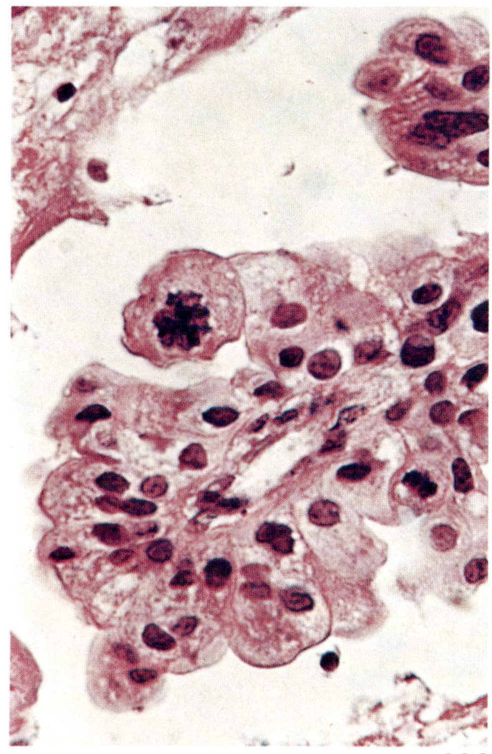

Fig. 6-4-1 (625×)
Patient A. S.C.S.F. Oligodendroglioma. The cytoplasm is pink.
The nuclei are round or oval and have no perinuclear halo.
There is a modest anisokaryosis and slight autolysis. The whole field is
monotone.

Fig. 6-4-2 (625×)
Same patient as in fig. 6-4-1. S.C.S.F. Oligodendroglioma.
A sheet of tumor cells with more pronounced crowding of nuclei.

Fig. 6-4-3 (400×)
Same patient as in fig. 6-4-1. Same S.C.S.F. preparation. Oligodendroglioma.
Here, the cytoplasm is basophil and there is maximal crowding of nuclei with
clumping of chromatin.

Fig. 6-4-4 (150×)
Same patient as in fig. 6-4-1. S.C.S.F. Oligodendroglioma.
Typical picture of oligodendroglioma in this overview.

6-4-1

6-4-2

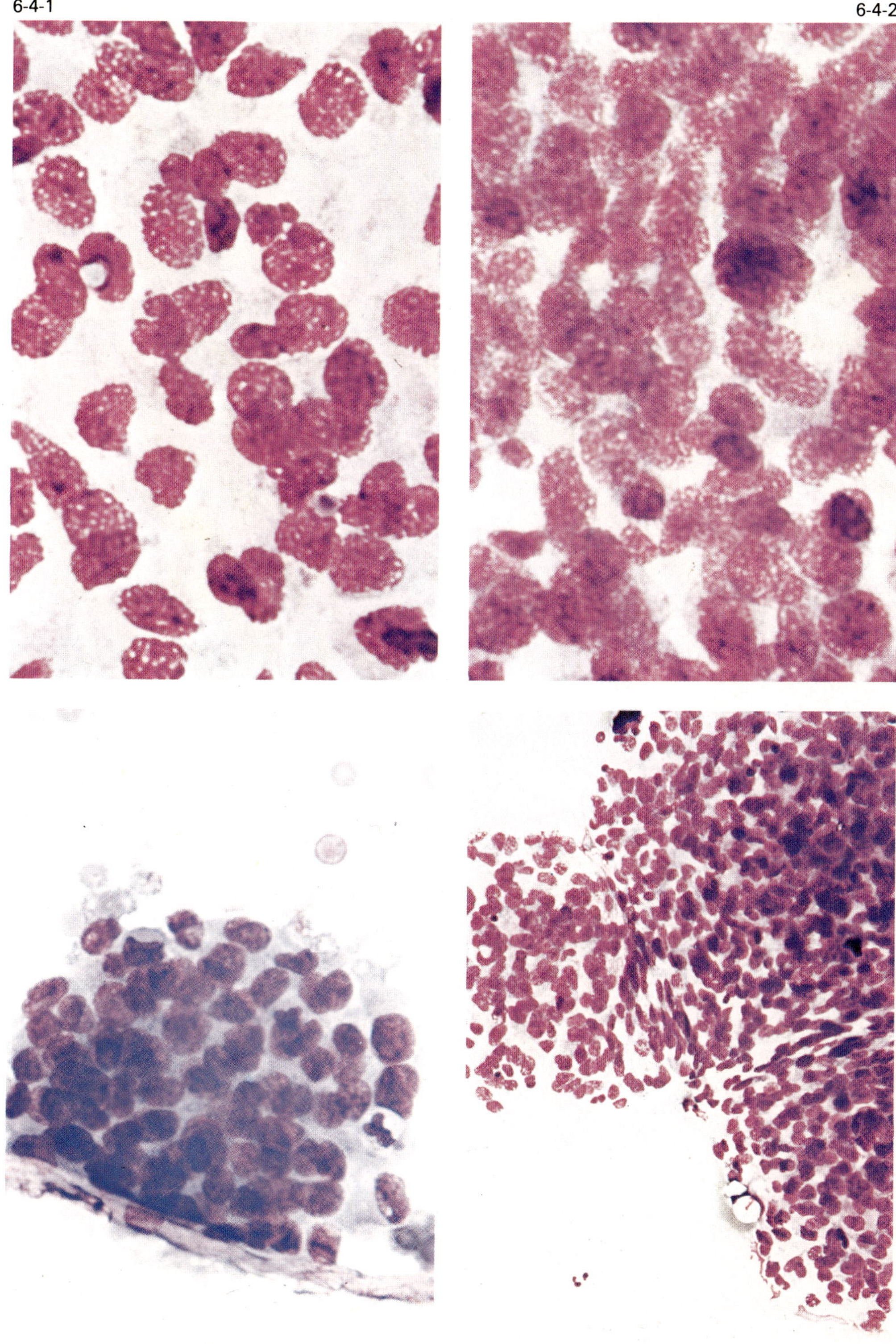

6-4-3

6-4-4

Fig. 6-4-5 (625 ×)
Same patient as in fig. 6-4-1. S.C.S.F. Oligodendroglioma.
In this tissue sheet less crowding of nuclei and only a modest anisokaryosis.
The cytoplasm is light blue.

Fig. 6-4-6 (625 ×)
Same patient as in fig. 6-4-1. S.C.S.F. Oligodendroglioma. Rosette formation.

Fig. 6-4-7 (400 ×)
Patient M. S.C.S.F. Oligodendroglioma. The nuclei are hyperchromatic.
There is some clumping of chromatin. The overall picture is monotone but the
nuclei are crowded.

Fig. 6-4-8 (400 ×)
Patient A. Oligodendroglioma. Smear preparation.
Resemblance with the C.S.F. preparations. Jenner–Giemsa staining.

6-4-5

6-4-6

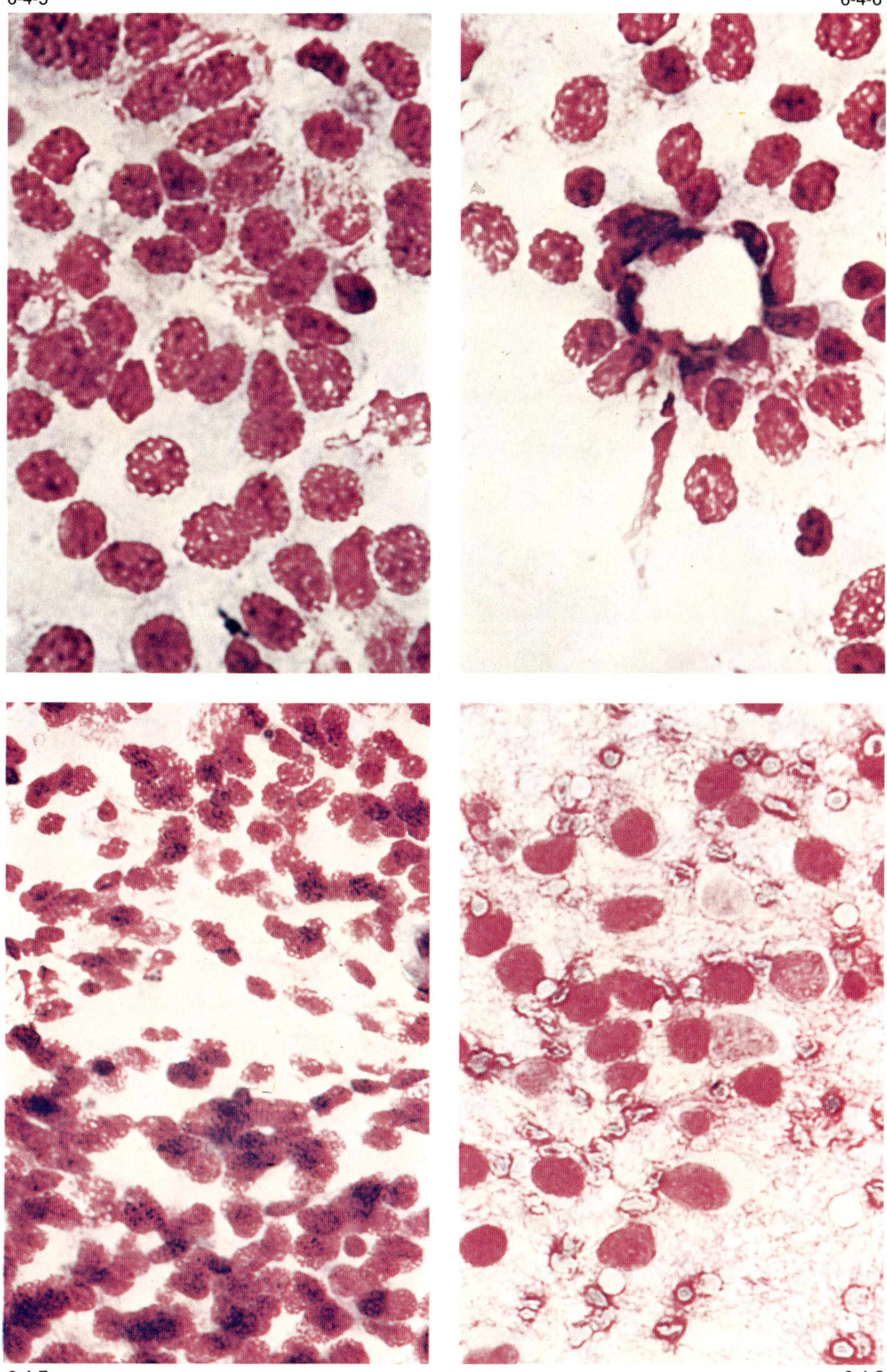

6-4-7

6-4-8

Fig. 6-4-9 (400×)
Same patient as in fig. 6-4-8. Oligodendroglioma. Smear preparation.
There is some anisokaryosis and the nuclei are more dispersed.
Jenner—Giemsa staining.

Fig. 6-5-1 (625×)
Patient v.L. S.C.S.F. Pinealoma. Large epitheloid cells with light-blue cytoplasm.
Marked polymorphism of the nuclei.

Fig. 6-5-2 (625×)
Same patient as in fig. 6-5-1. S.C.S.F. Pinealoma.
Same characteristics as in fig. 6-5-1. The cells are smaller.
The nuclei are hyperchromatic.

Fig. 6-5-3 (625×)
Same patient as in fig. 6-5-1. S.C.S.F. Pinealoma. Anisokaryosis.
Chromatin clumping.

6-4-9

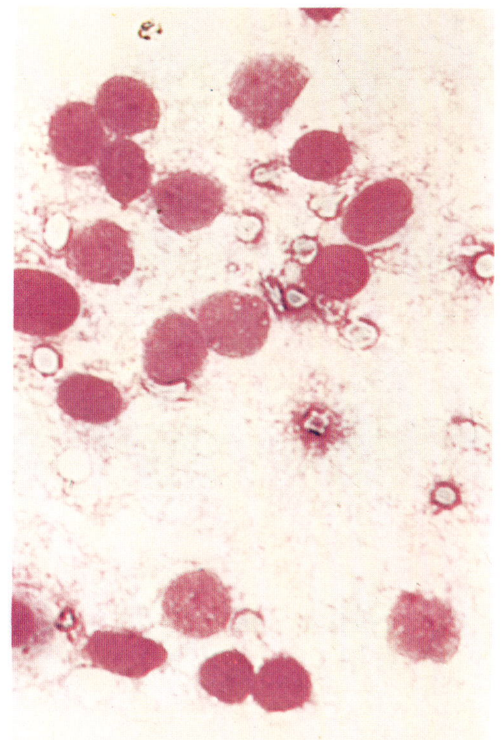

6-5-1

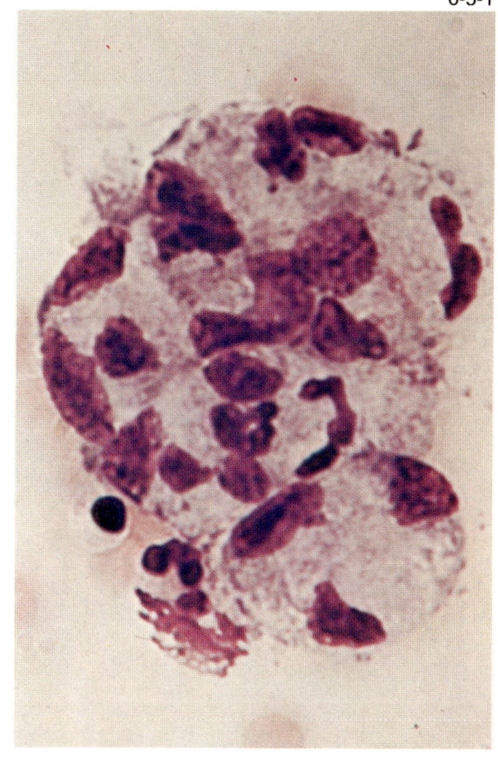

6-5-2

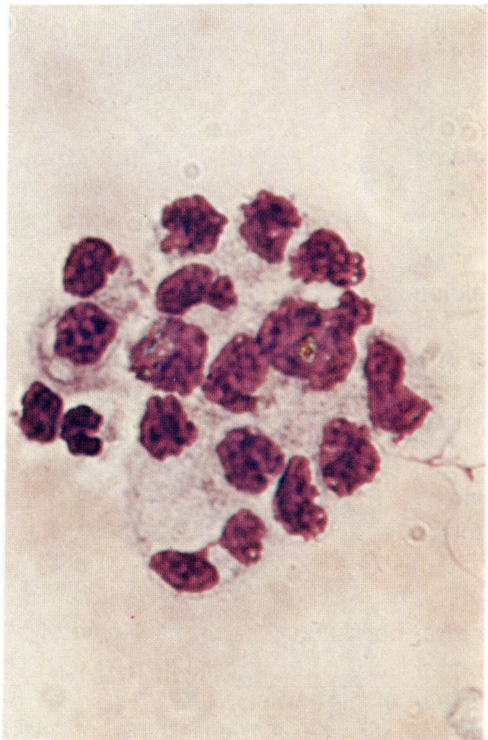

6-5-3

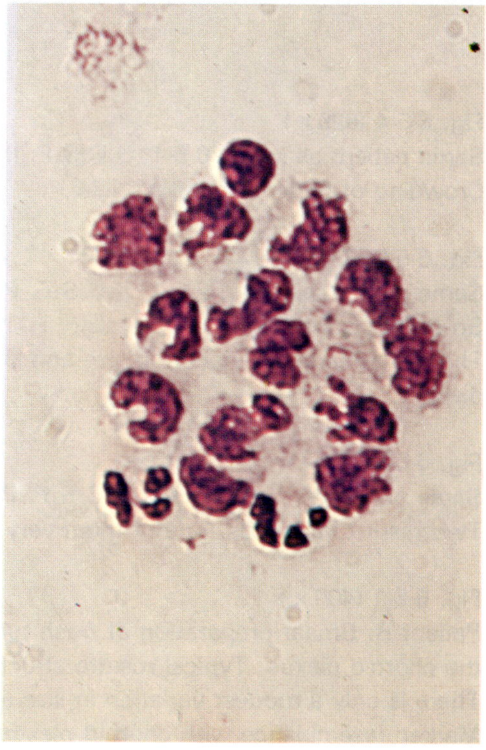

Fig. 6-6-2 (400 ×)
Patient B. Smear preparation. Benign papilloma of the choroid plexus. Here, the nuclei are more rounded.

Fig. 6-6-3 (400 ×)
Patient B. Smear preparation. Benign papilloma of the choroid plexus.
The peripheral nuclei are rather small in this specimen. No choroid plexus cells were found in the C.S.F. of this patient.

Fig. 6-7-1 (625 ×)
Patient K. Cyst aspirate. Chromophobe adenoma of the pituitary gland.
Distinct cell borders, pale red-violet cytoplasm, rounded nuclei.

Fig. 6-7-2 (625 ×)
Patient K. Cyst aspirate. Chromophobe adenoma of the pituitary gland.
The nuclei are slightly larger and show anisokaryosis.

6-6-2

6-6-3

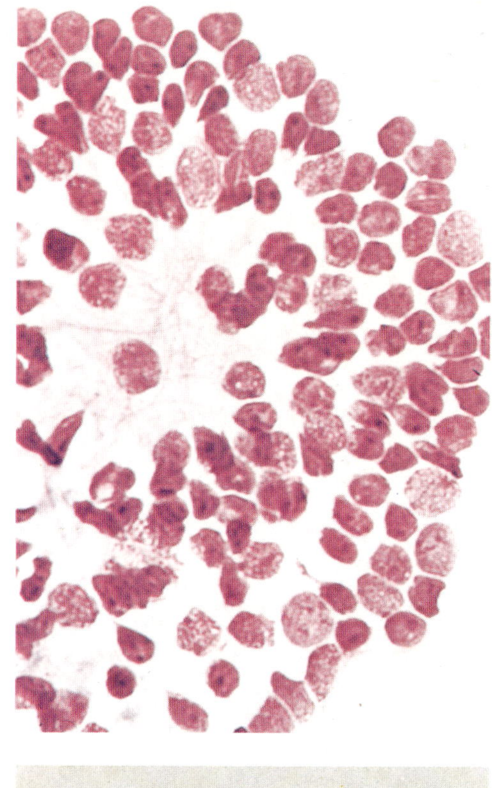

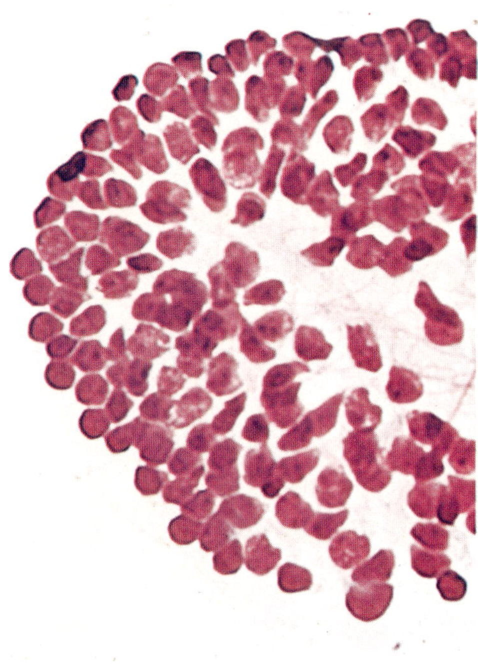

6-7-1

6-7-2

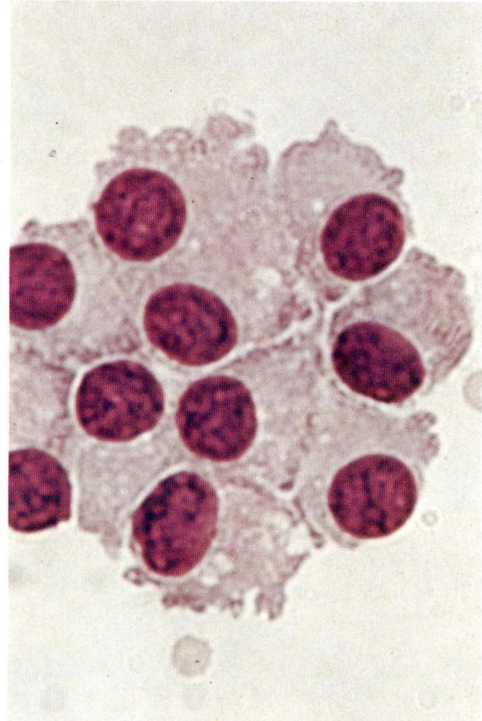

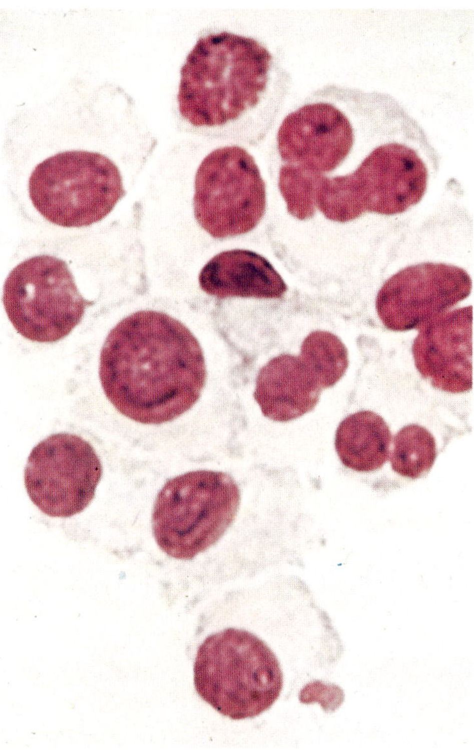

Fig. 6-7-3 (625 ×)
Patient U.-B. L.C.S.F. Chromophobe adenoma of the pituitary gland.
Tissue fragment. There is a perinuclear halo. The nuclei are pleomorph.
Distinct cell borders.

Fig. 6-7-4 (625 ×)
Patient U.-B. L.C.S.F. Chromophobe adenoma of the pituitary gland.
Tissue fragment with slight variation of size and shape of the nuclei.
The cell borders are less distinct.

Fig. 6-7-5 (625 ×)
Patient V.-v.I. Chromophobe adenoma of the pituitary gland.
Smear preparation. Typical rounded nuclei with anisokaryosis.

Fig. 6-8-1 (625 ×)
Patient V. Cyst aspirate. Eosinophil adenoma. The cytoplasm is eosinophil.
The nuclei are polymorph and hyperchromatic.

6-7-3

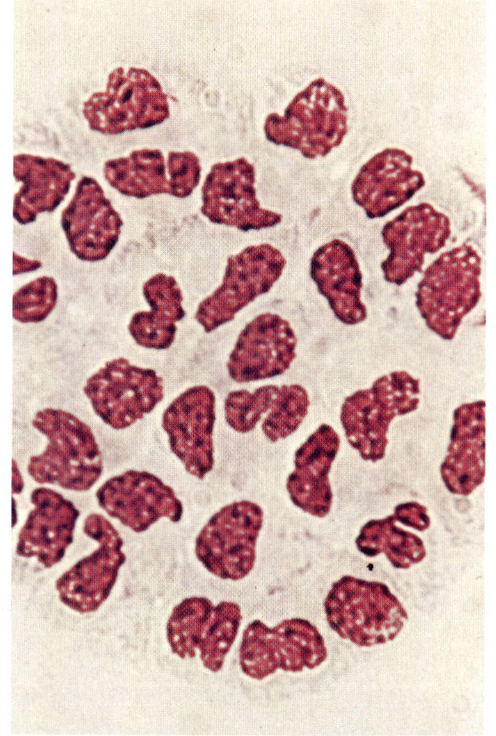

6-7-4

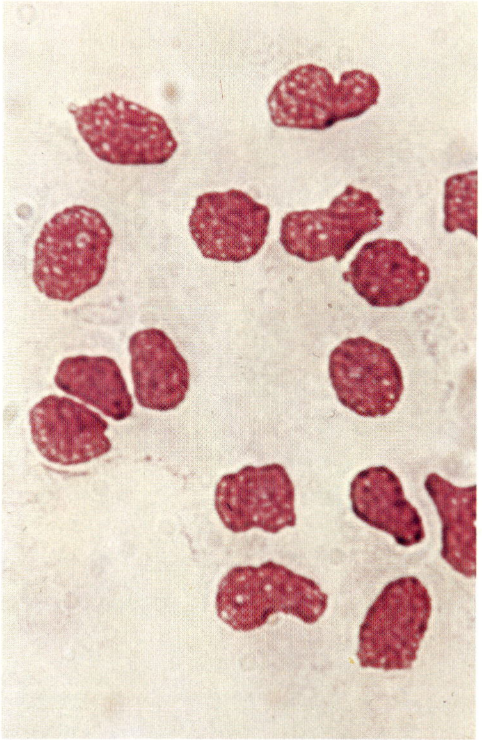

6-7-5

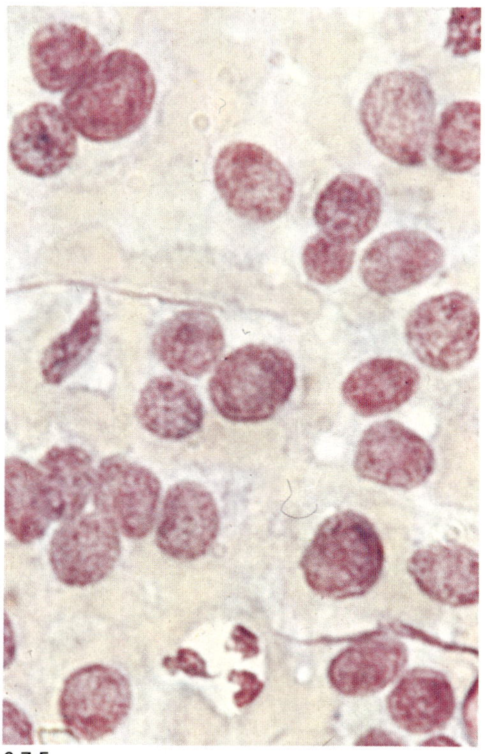

6-8-1

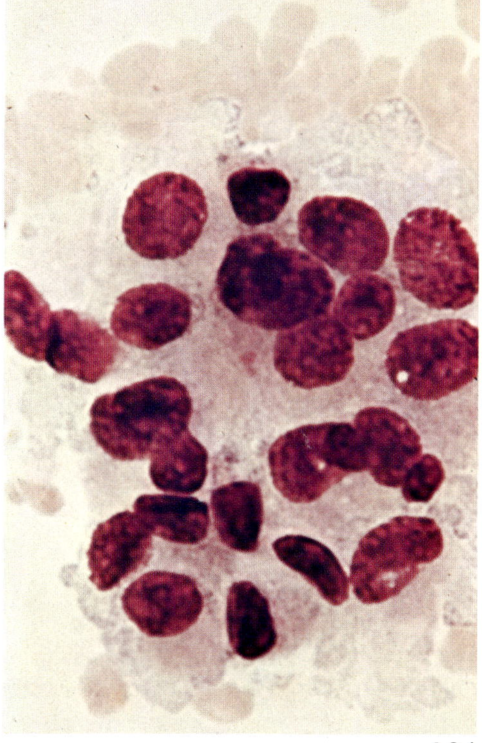

Fig. 6-8-2 (625×)
Patient V. Cyst aspirate. Eosinophil adenoma.
More pronounced anisokaryosis. Rosette structure. Hyperchromasia of the
nuclei.

Fig. 6-9-1 (400×)
Patient W. Craniopharyngeoma. Cyst aspirate.
Large group of small isomorph nuclei. The cytoplasm is light violet.

Fig. 6-9-2 (400×)
Patient R. Craniopharyngeoma. Cyst aspirate.
Group of the other type of craniopharyngeoma cells.
The nuclei are larger. The cytoplasm is light blue.

Fig. 6-9-3 (400×)
Patient W. Craniopharyngeoma. Cyst aspirate.
Both types of craniopharyngeoma cells in one picture.

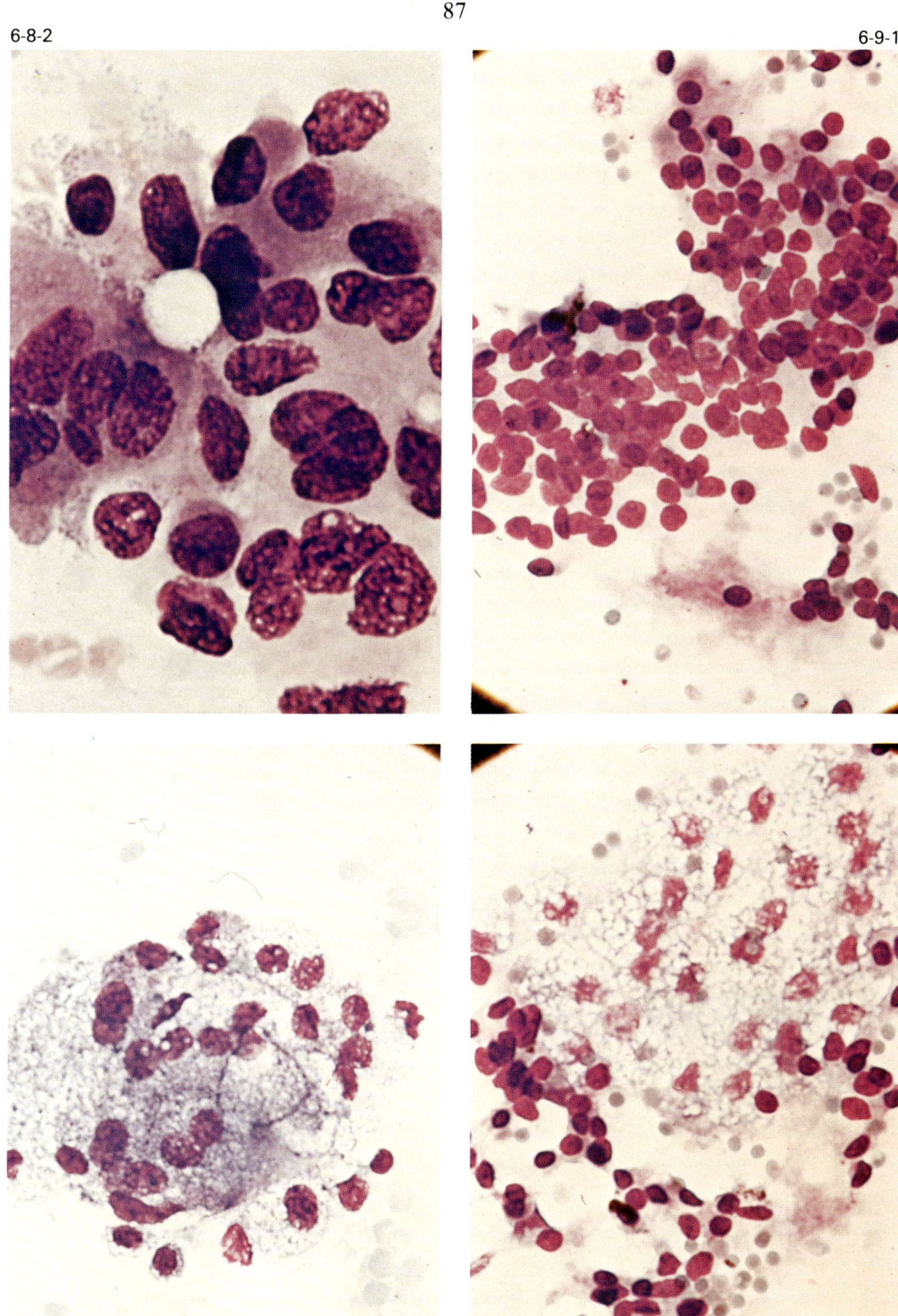
6-8-2
6-9-1
6-9-2
6-9-3

Fig. 6-9-4 (400×)
Patient B. Craniopharyngeoma. L.C.S.F. Tissue fragment with the same
characteristics as in fig. 6-9-2.

Fig. 6-9-5 (400×)
Patient B. Craniopharyngeoma. L.C.S.F. Another tissue sheet with slight
crowding of otherwise inactive nuclei.

Fig. 6-10-1 (100×)
Patient L. V.C.S.F. Middle ridge meningeoma. Fibrillar meningeoma.
Fragment of tumor tissue.

Fig. 6-10-2 (400×)
Patient K. S.C.S.F. Posterior fossa meningeoma. Endotheliomatous
meningeoma. Very marked crowding of nuclei. The cytoplasm is blue.

6-9-4

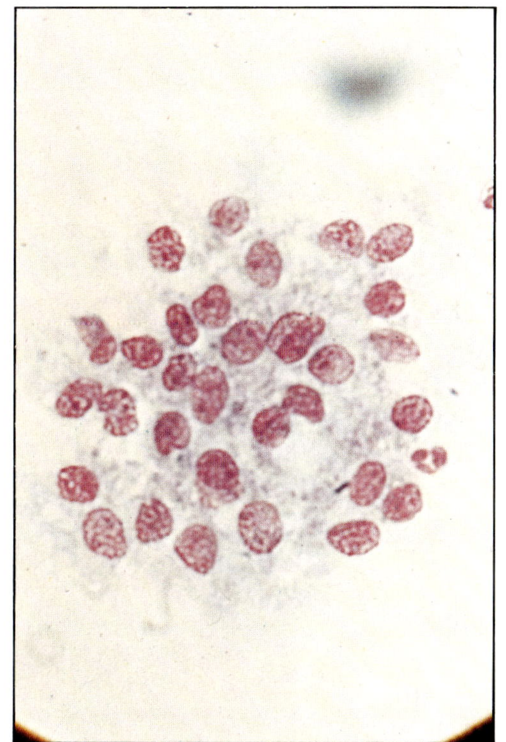

6-9-5

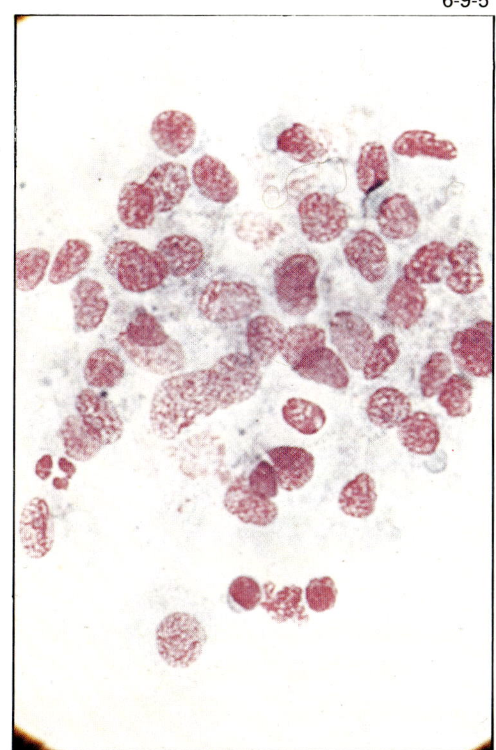

6-10-1

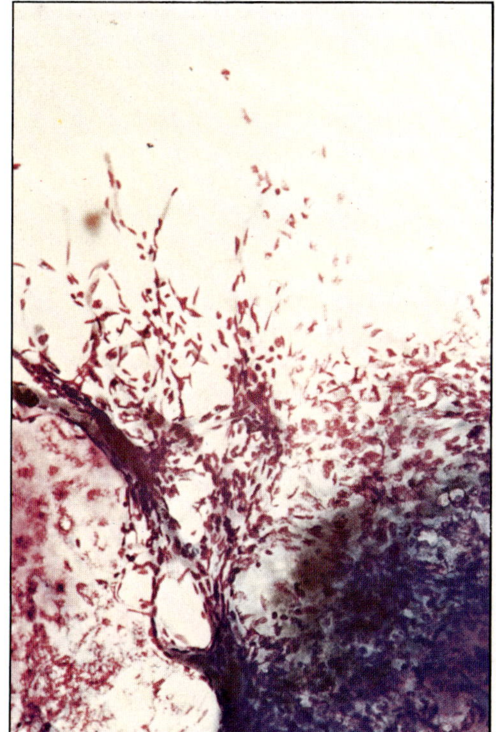

6-10-2

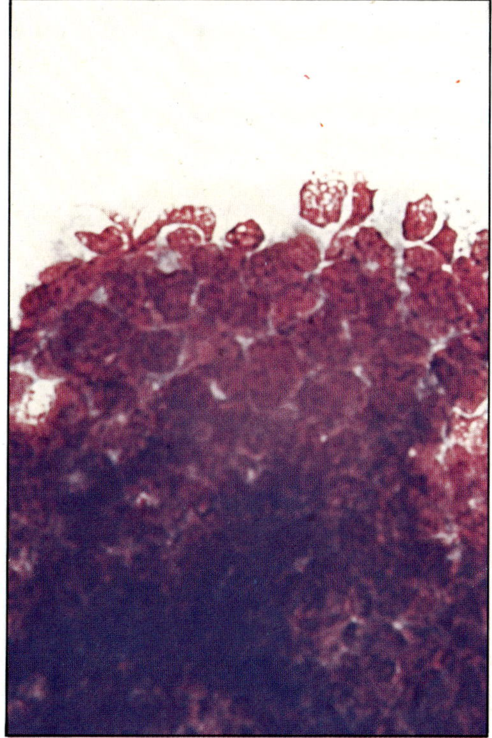

Fig. 6-10-3 (625×)
Patient V. L.C.S.F. Falx meningeoma. Endotheliomatous meningeoma.
Strong resemblance with arachnoidea. There is more pleomorphism than in
arachnoidea. Spinal tap 3 days after incomplete ablation of tumor.
Irregular nuclear contours.

Fig. 6-10-4 (625×)
Same patient as in fig. 6-10-3. L.C.S.F. Falx meningeoma. Endotheliomatous
meningeoma. An other cluster of tumor cells. Marked difference in size and
shape of nuclei.

Fig. 6-10-5 (625×)
Same patient as in fig. 6-10-3. L.C.S.F. Falx meningeoma. Endotheliomatous
meningeoma. A cluster of tumor cells with less crowding of nuclei.

Fig. 6-10-6 (625×)
Same patient as in fig. 6-10-3. L.C.S.F. Falx meningeoma. Endotheliomatous
meningeoma. Marked polymorphism of the nuclei and more crowding.
The cytoplasm of the cells is light-blue. The cell borders are clearly visible.

6-10-3

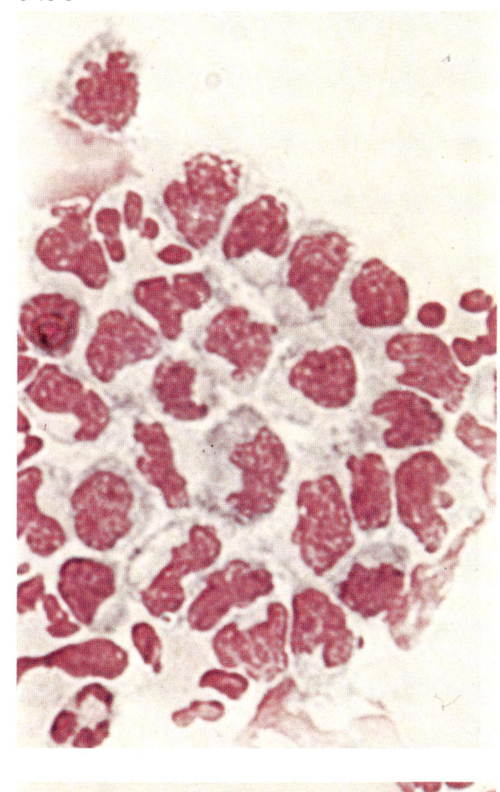

6-10-4

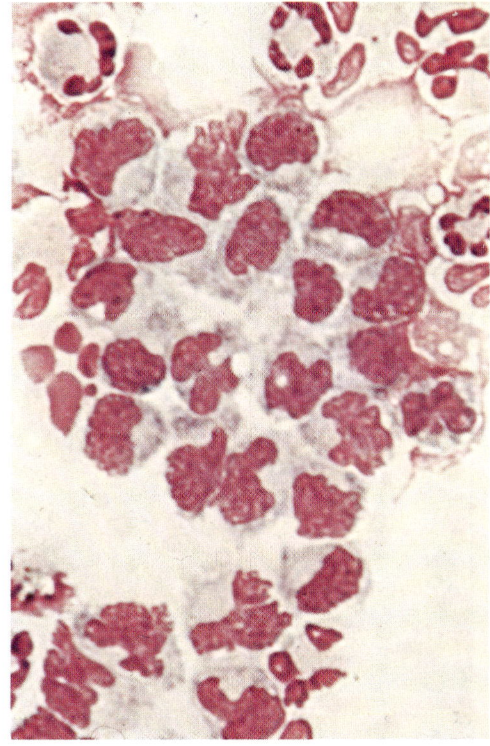

6-10-5

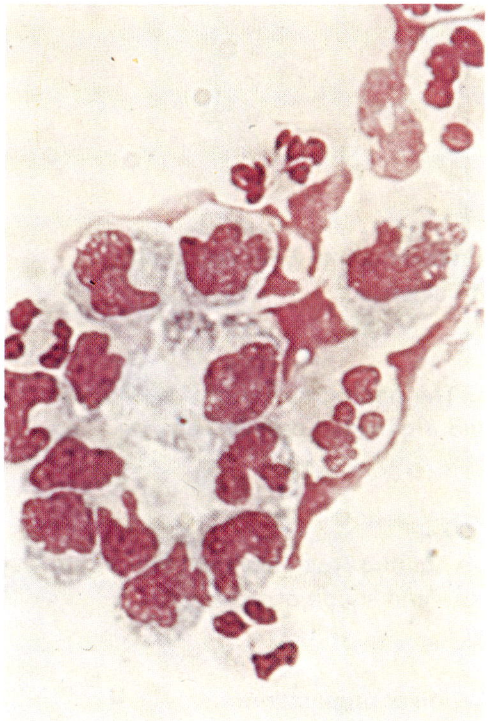

6-10-6

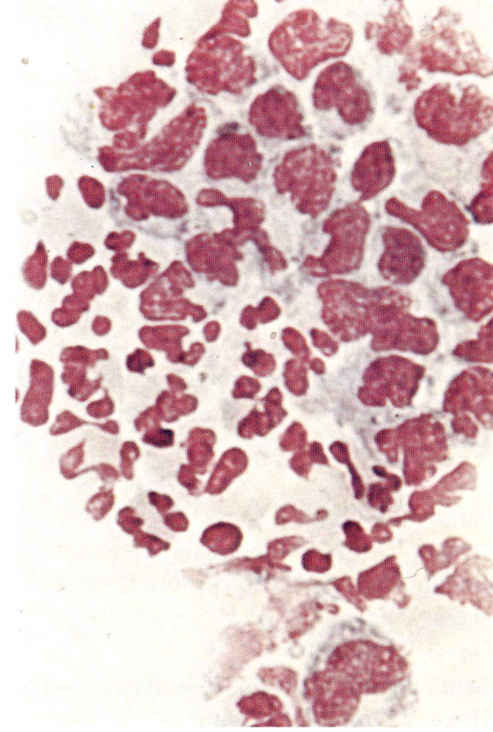

Fig. 6-11-1 (250×)
Patient v.B. L.C.S.F. Left-sided acoustic neurinoma.
The fibrillar sometimes whorling structure of the tissue stroma is evident.
The nuclei are not isomorph. This is a preparation from a lumbar puncture a day
after the operation and shows spreading of this benign tumor in the C.S.F.

Fig. 6-11-2 (400×)
Same patient as in fig. 6-11-1. L.C.S.F. Left-sided acoustic neurinoma.
Marked fibrillar structure of the stroma and anisomorph nuclei.

Fig. 6-11-3 (400×)
Same patient as in fig. 6-11-1. L.C.S.F. Left-sided acoustic neurinoma.
Same picture as fig. 6-11-1 but less crowding of nuclei.

Fig. 6-12-1 (625×)
Patient M. L.C.S.F. Colloid cyst, third ventricle. Tissue fragment with violet-
colored cytoplasm and slight polymorphism and hyperchromasia of the nuclei.
There is some resemblance with normal ependyma or choroid plexus from which
the colloid cyst originates.

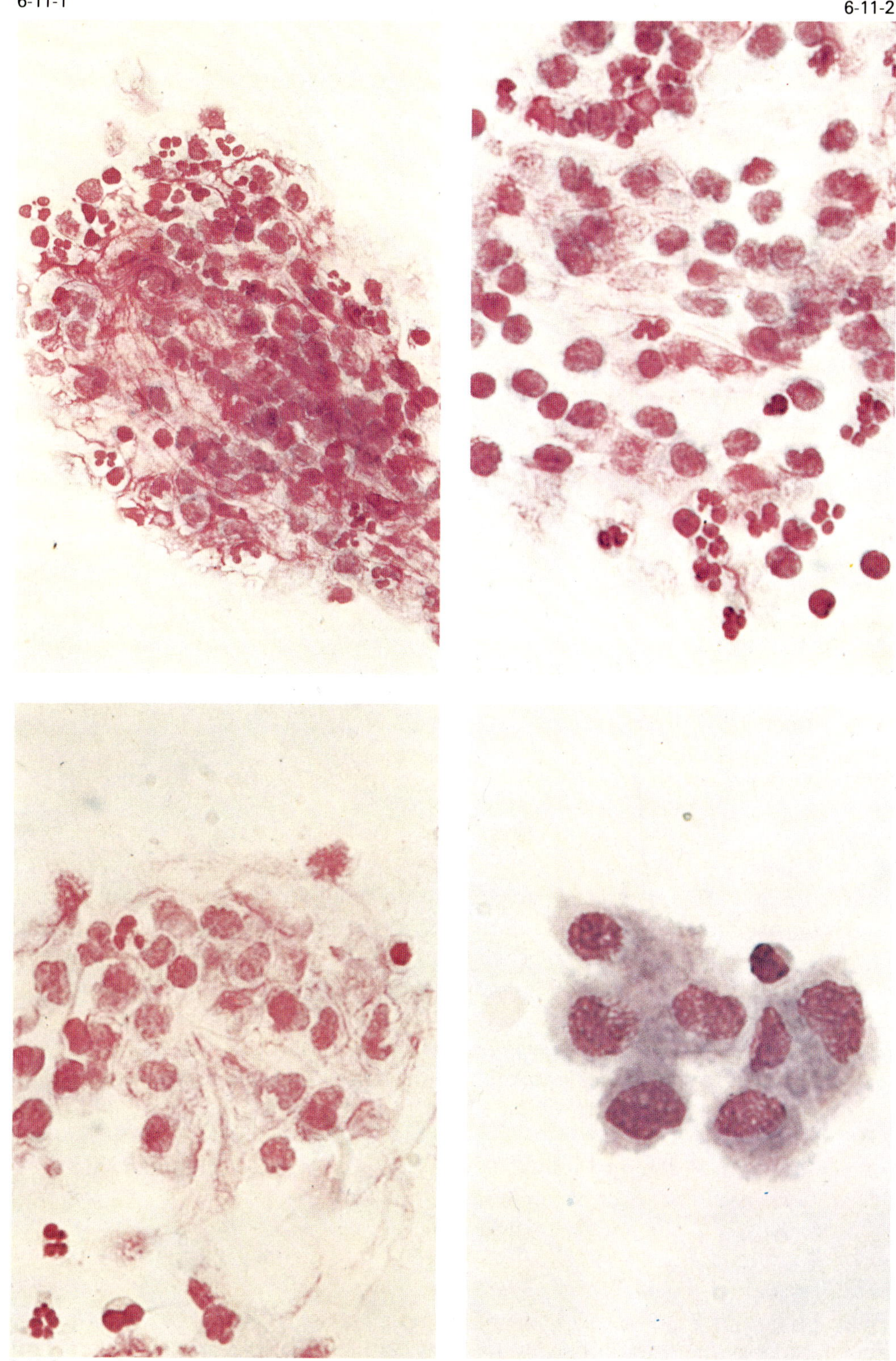
6-11-1
6-11-2
6-11-3
6-12-1

Fig. 7-1-1 (400 ×)
Patient Sj. S.C.S.F. Squamous carcinoma of the lung with transverse lesion.
Large tumor fragment with bizarre nuclei and a fine granulation in the cytoplasm
(keratin). This is the squamous type with cornification (keratin formation).

Fig. 7-1-2 (625 ×)
Patient W. L.C.S.F. Squamous carcinoma of the lung with transverse lesion.
Isolated keratin-containing cell in mitosis. Metastasis. Cerebellar angle tumor.

Fig. 7-1-3 (625 ×)
Patient W. L.C.S.F. Cerebellar angle tumor. Squamous carcinoma of the lung.
Metastasis. Tissue fragment of tumor cells. Crowding of nuclei.
Marked variation in size and shape of the nuclei.

Fig. 7-1-4 (625 ×)
Patient W. L.C.S.F. Cerebellar angle tumor. Squamous carcinoma of the lung.
Tissue fragment of tumor cells with the same characteristics as fig. 7-1-3.

7-1-1

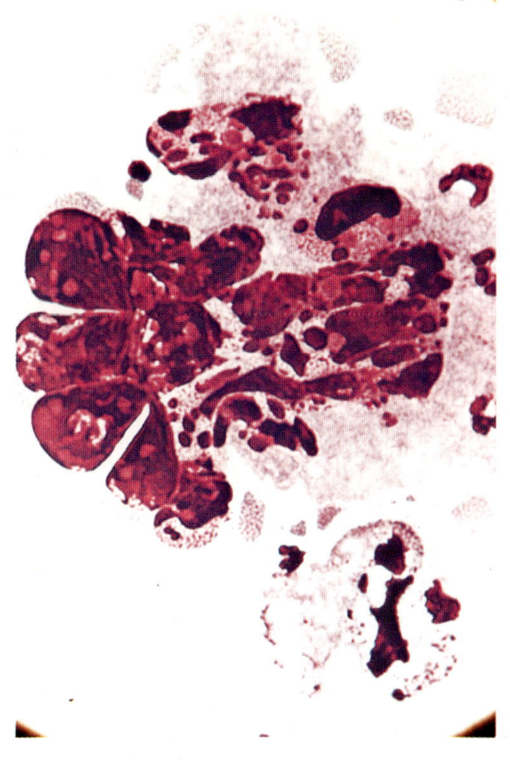

7-1-2

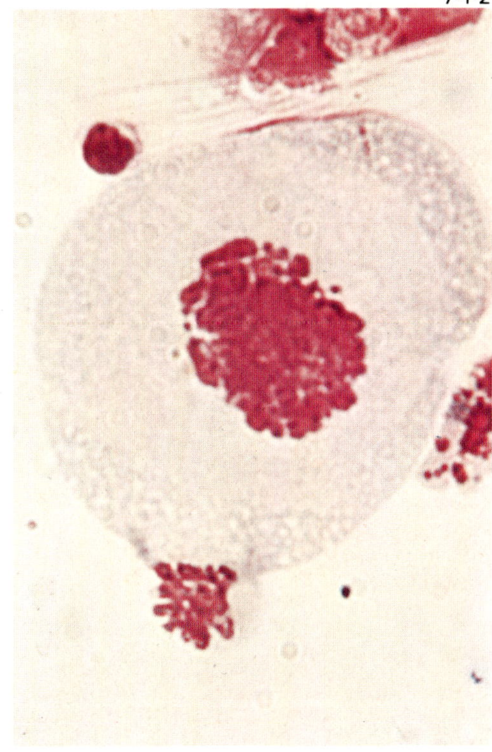

7-1-3

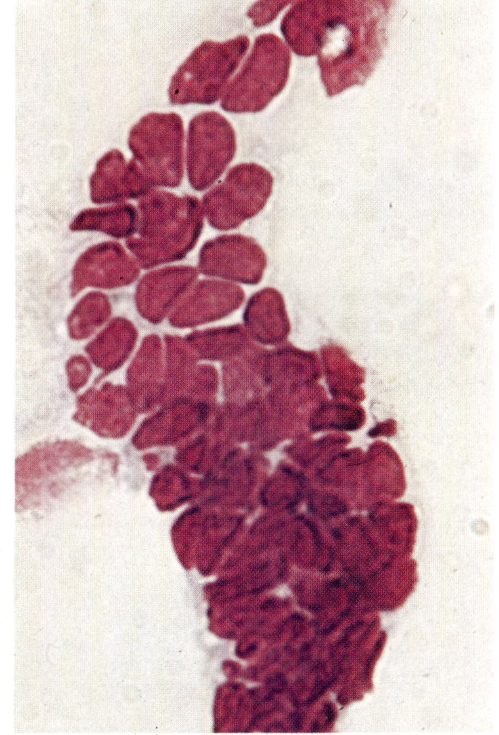

7-1-4

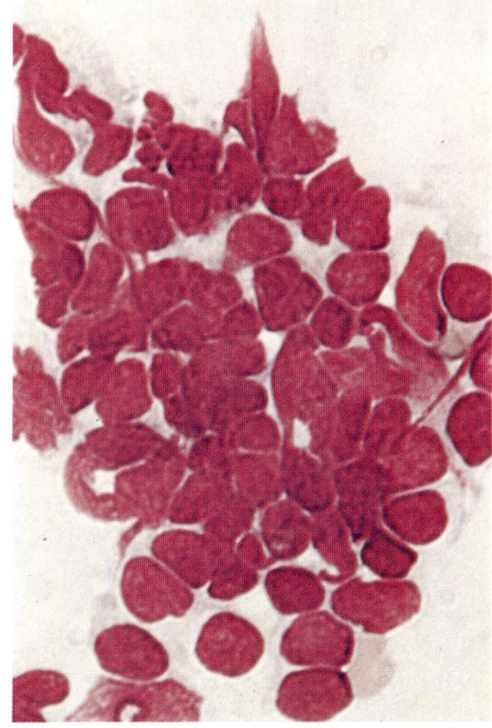

Fig. 7-1-5 (625×)
Patient W. L.C.S.F. Cerebellar angle tumor. Squamous carcinoma of the lung.
Small cluster of tumor cells. The cytoplasm has the typical color of the
squamous carcinoma cell.

Fig. 7-1-6 (625×)
Patient W. L.C.S.F. Cerebellar angle tumor. Squamous carcinoma of the lung.
Giant tumor cell with relatively small nucleus. Another tumor cell has a larger
nucleus and smaller cell size.

Fig. 7-1-7 (625×)
Patient W. L.C.S.F. Cerebellar angle tumor. Squamous carcinoma of the lung.
Tumor cells with prominent nucleoli and blue cytoplasm.

Fig. 7-1-8 (625×)
Patient W. L.C.S.F. Cerebellar angle tumor. Squamous carcinoma of the lung.
Tumor cells with anisocytosis, anisokaryosis and the typical cytoplasm of the
keratinizing type of tumor. Very prominent nucleoli. Irregular nuclear contours.

7-1-5

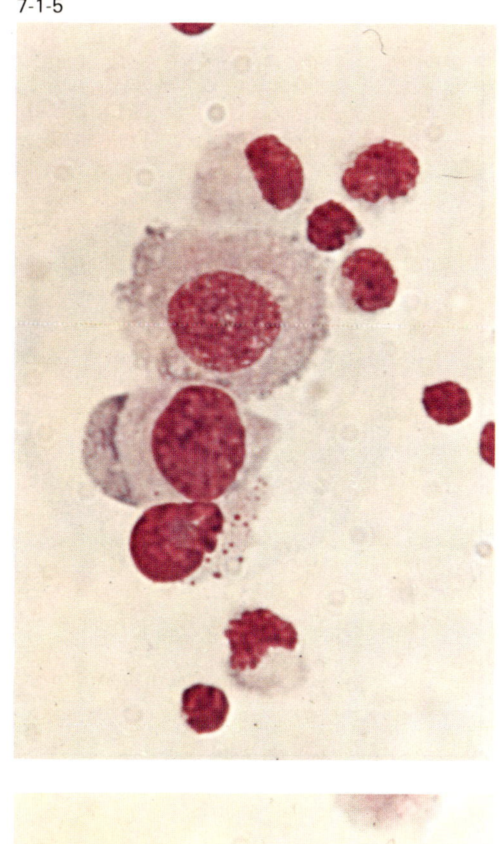

7-1-6

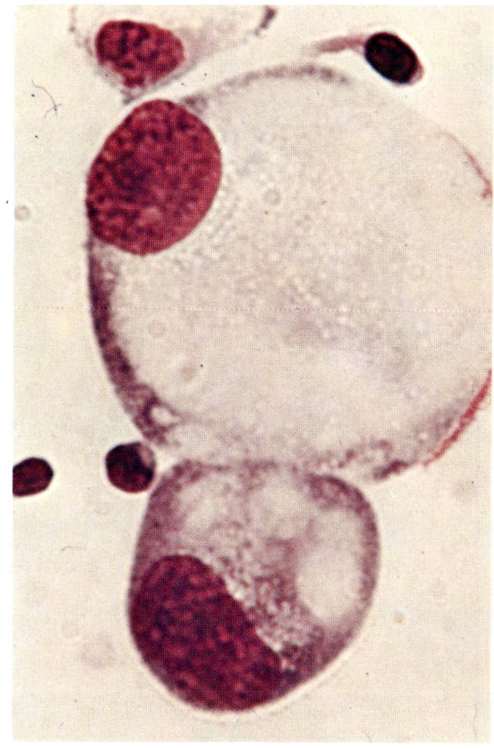

7-1-7

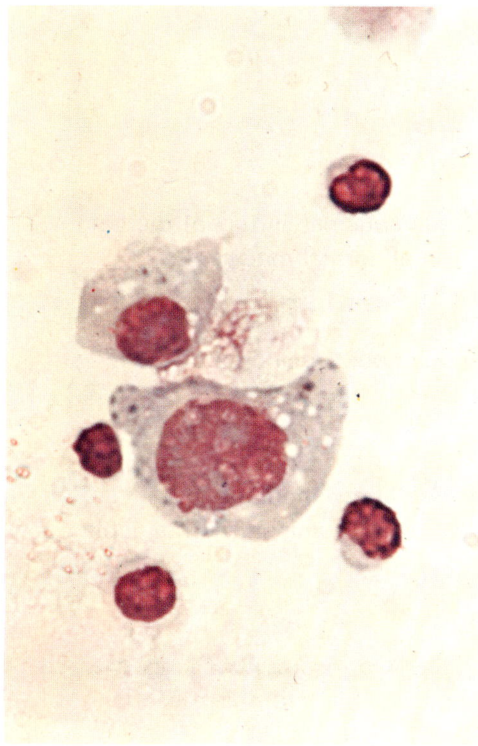

7-1-8

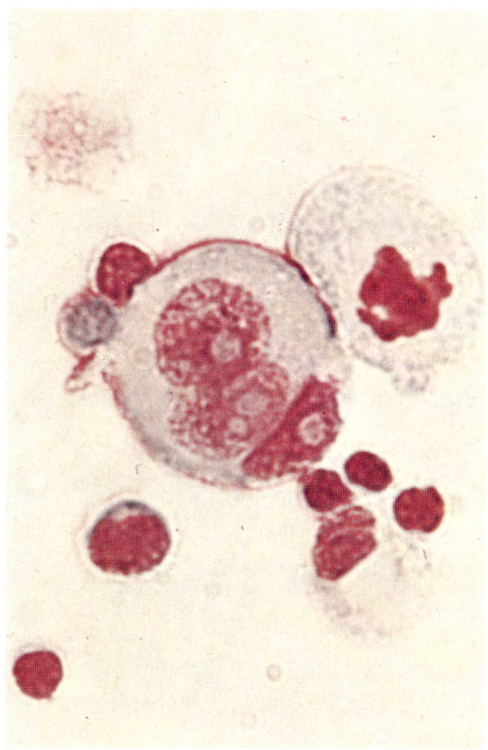

Fig. 7-2-3 (625 ×)
Patient L.v.I. L.C.S.F. Carcinomatous meningitis. Adenocarcinoma lung.
Marked anisocytosis and anisokaryosis. Blue-violet granulated cytoplasm.
Distinct cell borders. Prominent nucleoli.

Fig. 7-2-4 (625 ×)
Patient L.v.I. L.C.S.F. Carcinomatous meningitis. Adenocarcinoma lung.
Crowding of nuclei. High nucleus–cytoplasm ratio.
Marked anisokaryosis and pleomorphism.

Fig. 7-3-1 (400 ×)
Patient Sch. L.C.S.F. Carcinomatous meningitis. Carcinoma of the breast.
Group of tumor cells with anisocytosis and anisokaryosis. The cytoplasm is light-
blue. There is one large signet ring cell.

Fig. 7-3-2 (400 ×)
Same patient as fig. 7-3-1. L.C.S.F. Carcinomatous meningitis. Carcinoma of the
breast. Group of tumor cells, one of them very large. The cell borders are
distinct.

7-2-3

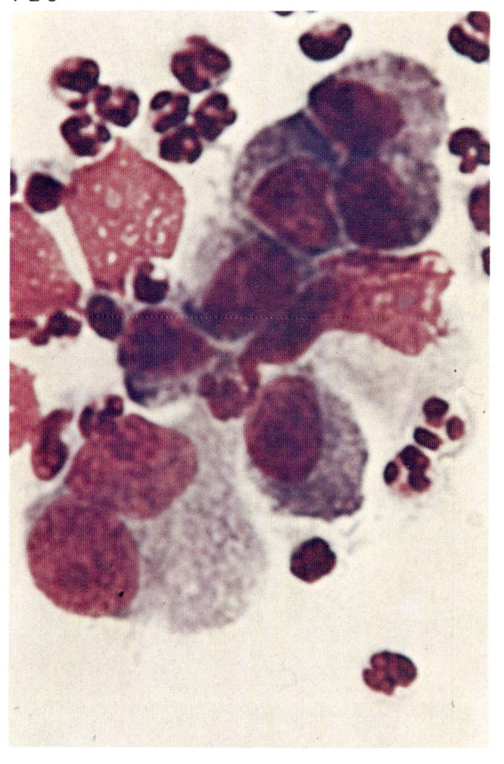

7-2-4

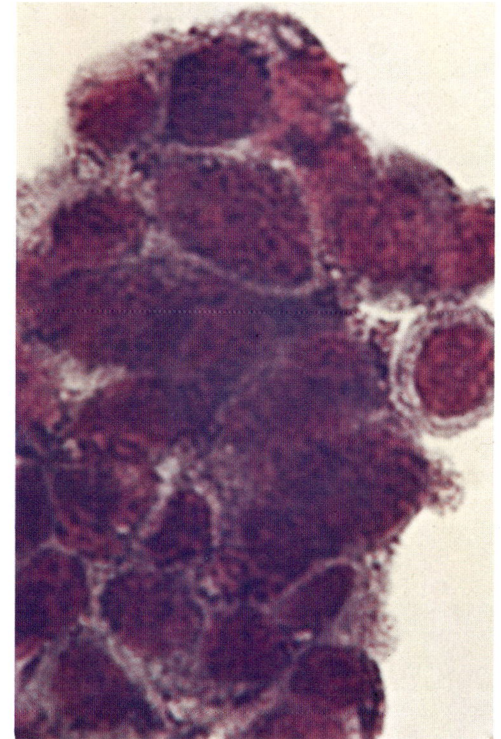

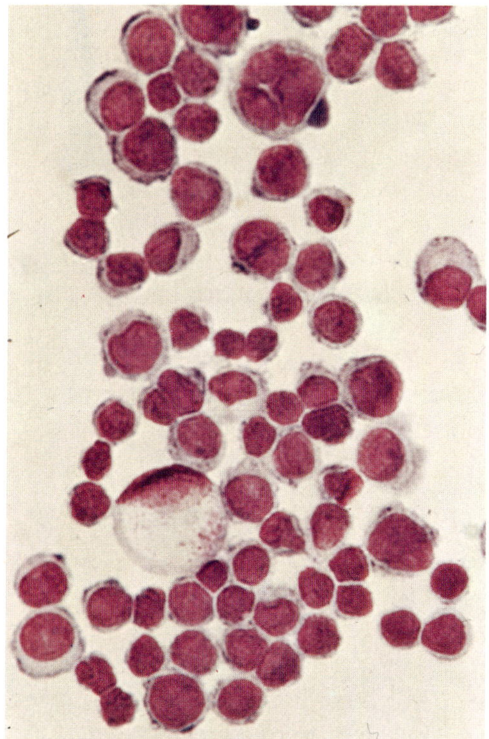

7-3-1

7-3-2

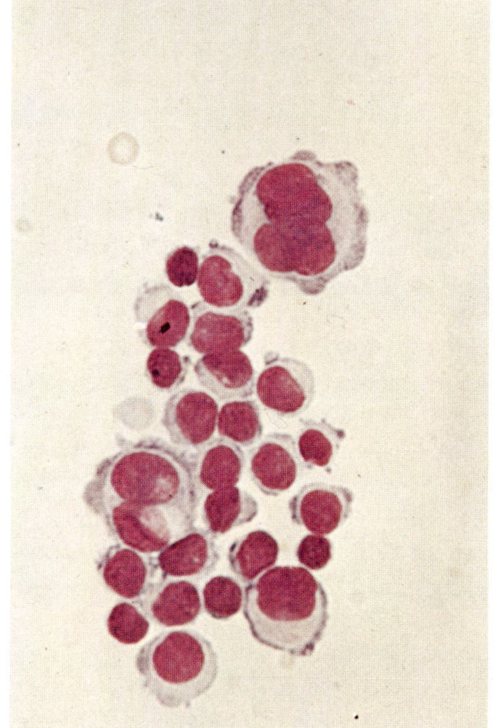

Fig. 7-3-3 (400×)
Same patient as fig. 7-3-1. L.C.S.F. Carcinomatous meningitis. Carcinoma of the breast. The numerous tumor cells point to meningeal carcinomatosis.

Fig. 7-3-4 (400×)
Same patient as fig. 7-3-1. L.C.S.F. Carcinomatous meningitis. Carcinoma of the breast. Group of tumor cells. There is one signet-ring cell and one cell with two nuclei. There is evident nuclear polymorphism.

Fig. 7-3-5 (400×)
Patient W.K. L.C.S.F. Carcinoma of the breast. Carcinoma solidum. The nuclei show hyperchromasia and anisokaryosis. There is anisocytosis.

Fig. 7-3-6 (400×)
Patient v.D. L.C.S.F. Carcinoma of the breast. Crowding of polymorph nuclei. Giant tumor cells. Multiple nuclei in one cell. Granulated dark-blue cytoplasm.

7-3-3

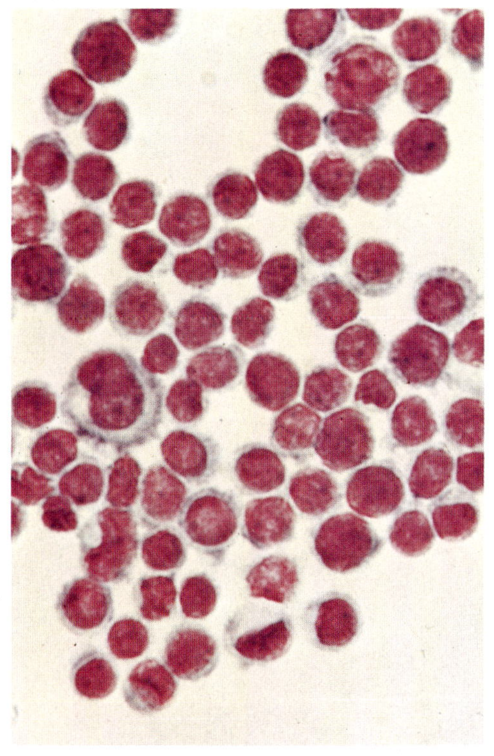

7-3-4

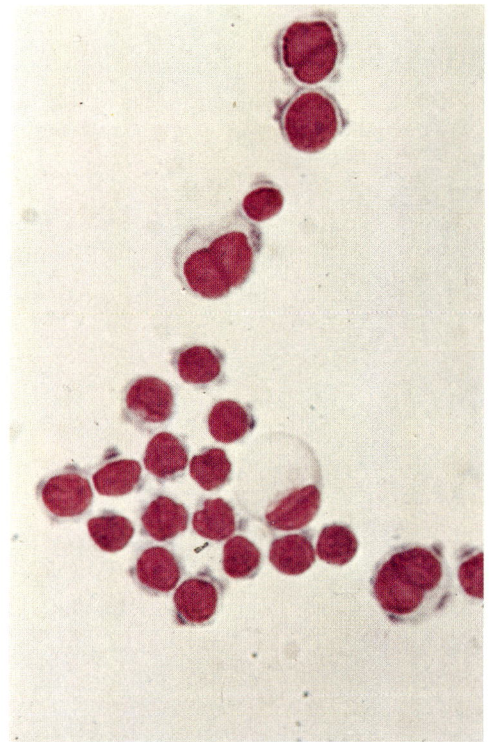

7-3-5

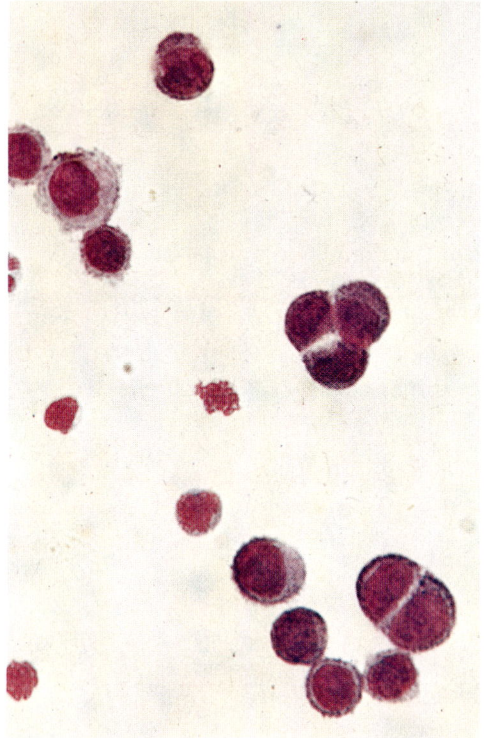

7-3-6

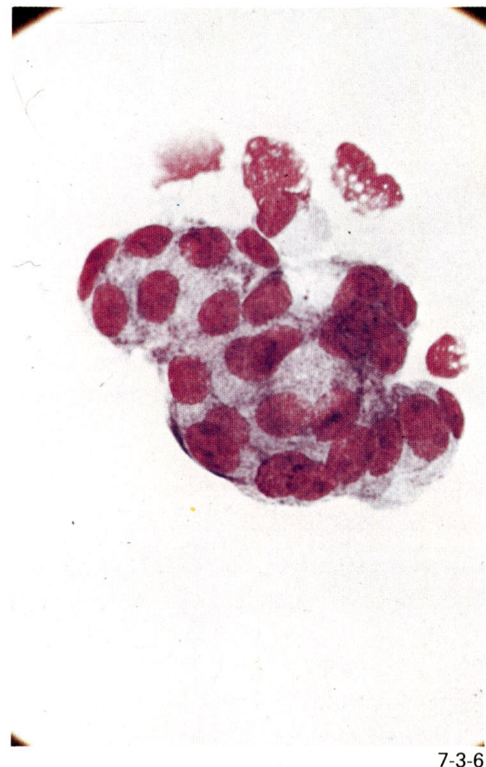

Fig. 7-3-7 (400 ×)
Patient v.D. Carcinoma of the breast. Papanicolaou staining.
The cell margins are even more distinct than in the Jenner–Giemsa staining.

Fig. 7-3-8 (400 ×)
Patient v.D. Carcinoma of the breast. Papanicolaou staining.
Papilliform structure of the tissue fragment of tumor cells.

Fig. 7-4-1 (400 ×)
Patient A. L.C.S.F. Carcinoma ventriculi.
The usual characteristics of a malignant tumor.
A tissue fragment of crowded nuclei with anisonucleosis.
The cytoplasm is blue-violet and granulated.

Fig. 7-4-2 (400 ×)
Same patient as in fig. 7-4-1. L.C.S.F. Carcinoma ventriculi.
Multiple nuclei in one cell. Two cells are of the signet ring type.

7-3-7

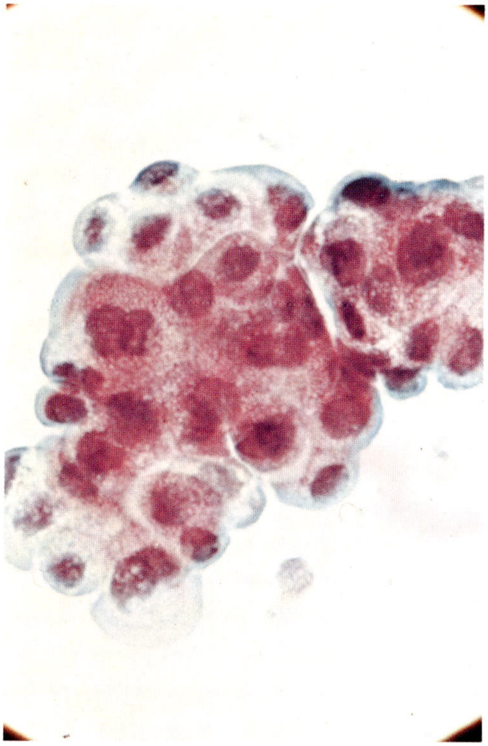

7-3-8

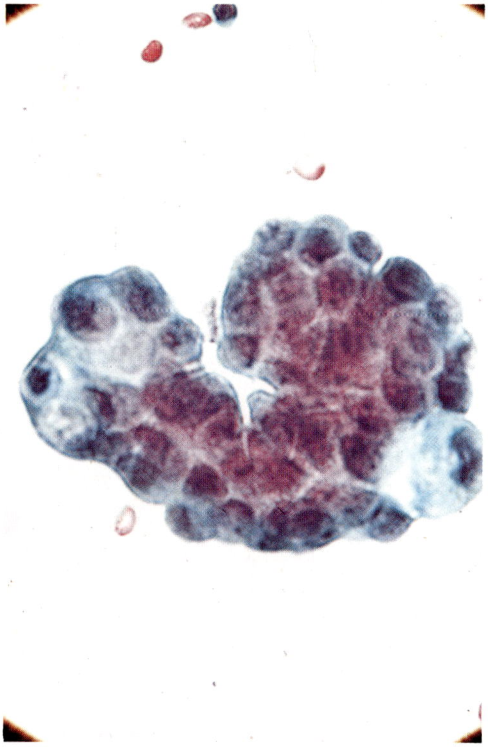

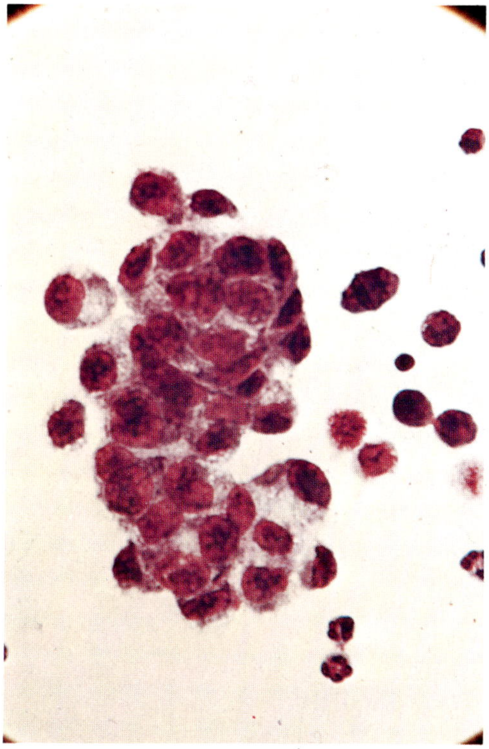

7-4-1

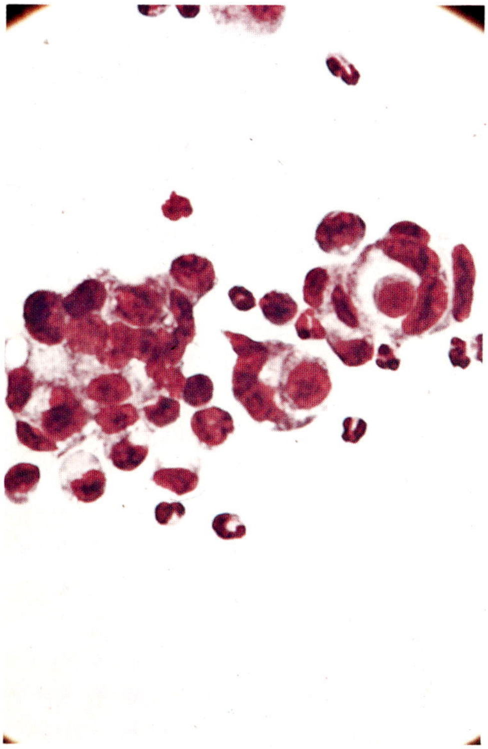

7-4-2

Fig. 7-4-3 (400×)
Same patient as in fig. 7-4-1. L.C.S.F. Carcinoma ventriculi.
Free lying tumor cells and signet ring cells.

Fig. 7-4-4 (400×)
Same patient as in fig. 7-4-1. L.C.S.F. Carcinoma ventriculi.
Marked polymorphism of cells and nuclei.

Fig. 7-4-5 (400×)
Patient F. L.C.S.F. Carcinoma ventriculi. The cells are larger than those in case
fig. 7-4-1. There are prominent nucleoli.

Fig. 7-4-6 (400×)
Same patient as in fig. 7-4-5. L.C.S.F. Carcinoma ventriculi.
Large tissue sheet. Same picture as in fig. 7-4-5.

7-4-3

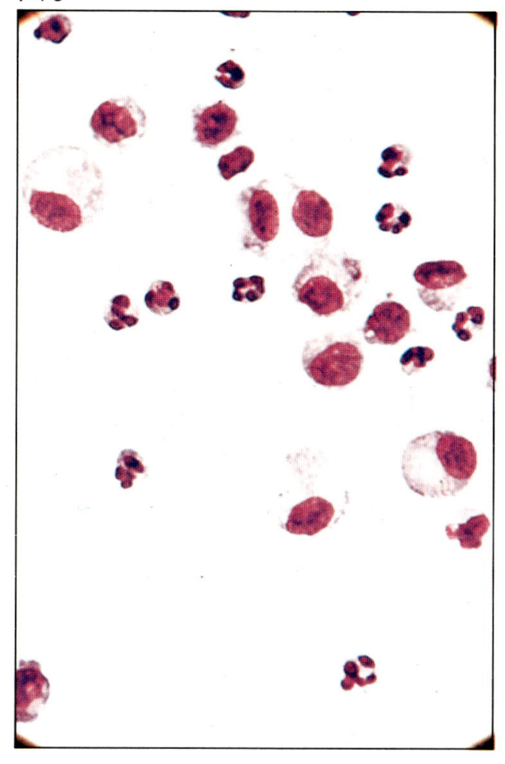

7-4-4

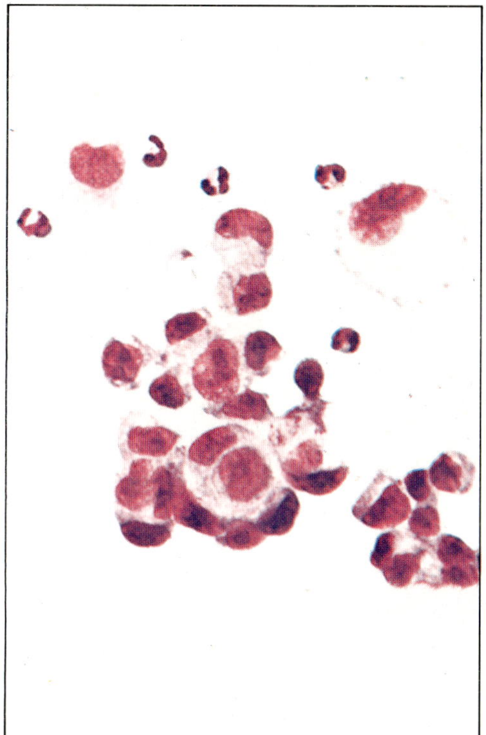

7-4-5

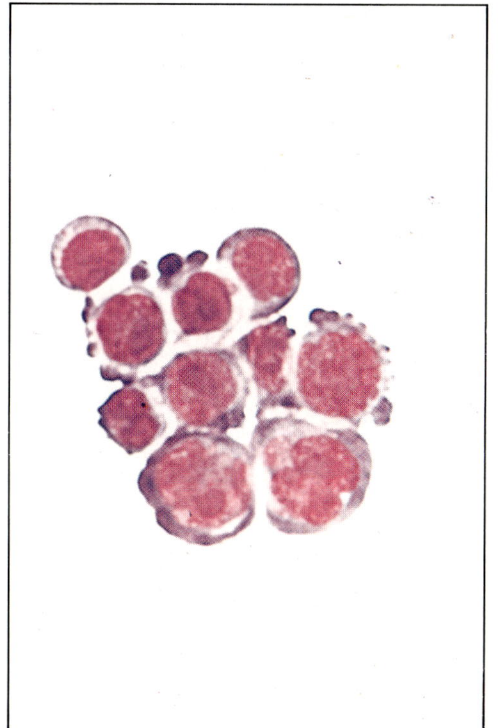

7-4-6

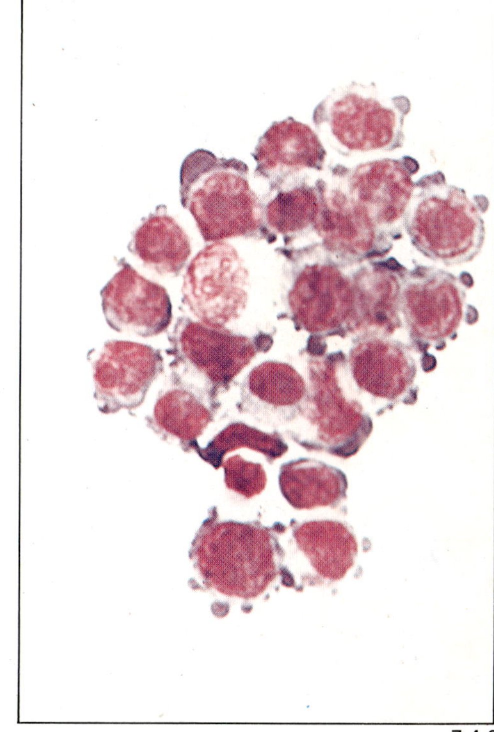

Fig. 7-4-7 (400 ×)
Same patient as in fig. 7-4-5. L.C.S.F. Carcinoma ventriculi.
The nucleus–cytoplasm ratio is strongly increased in favour of the nuclei.

Fig. 7-4-8 (400 ×)
Same patient as in fig. 7-4-5. L.C.S.F. Carcinoma ventriculi.
Free lying tumor cells of the same morphology as in the tissue fragment of
fig. 7-4-7.

Fig. 7-5-1 (400 ×)
Patient G. L.C.S.F. Carcinoma coli. A small tissue fragment of three cells.
The cytoplasm is light-blue. The cell contours distinct. The nuclei are polymorph
and their contours irregular. A differential diagnosis with carcinoma recti is
impossible.

Fig. 7-5-2 (400 ×)
Same patient as in fig. 7-5-1. L.C.S.F. Carcinoma coli.
One free lying tumor cell. This cell has phagocytized an erythrocyte. The nucleus
shows nuclear membrane irregularities.

Fig. 7-6-1 (400 ×)
Patient V. L.C.S.F. Carcinoma recti. Tissue sheet with cells with light-blue
cytoplasm and polymorphism of the nuclei.

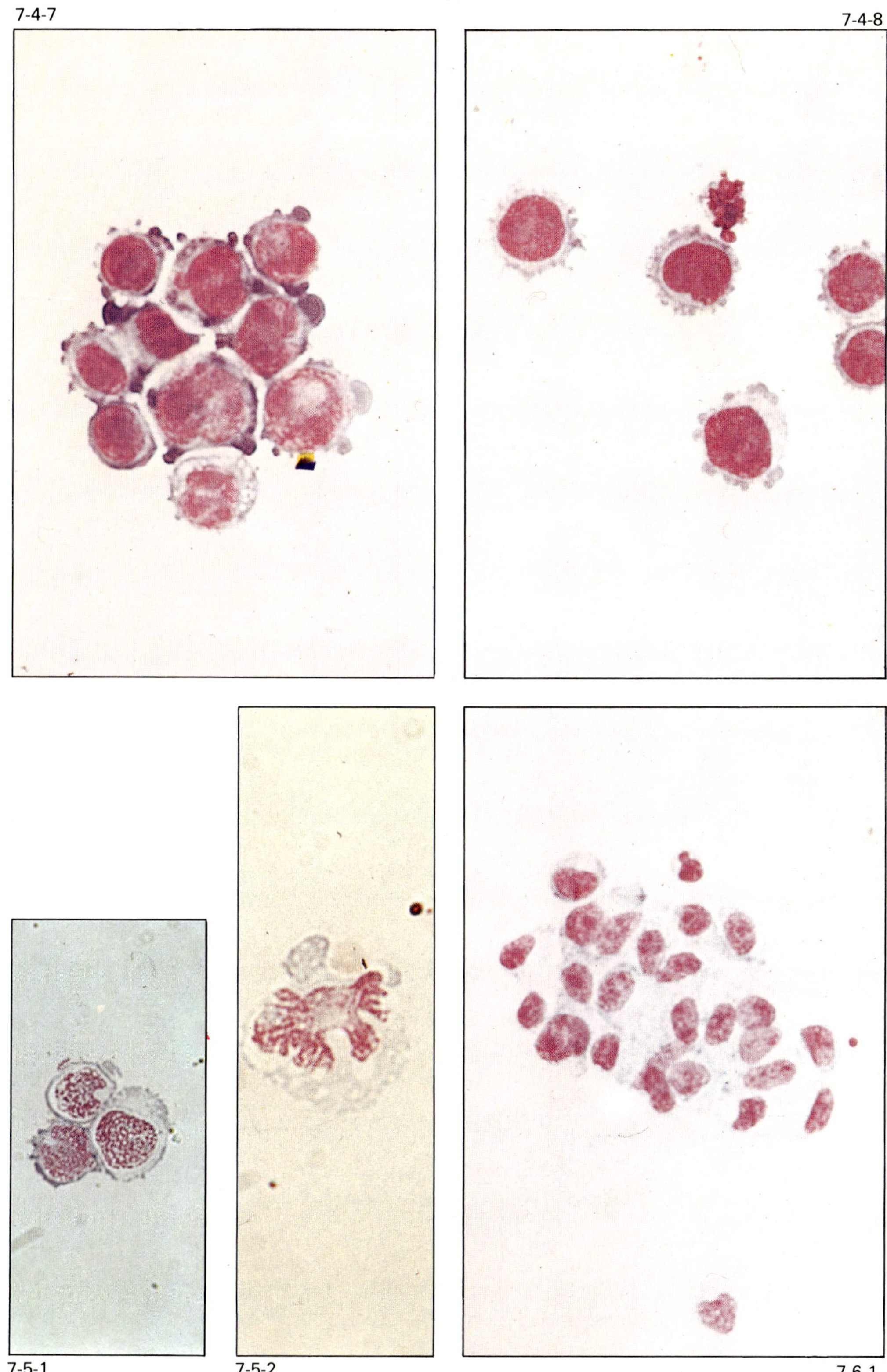
7-4-7
7-4-8
7-5-1
7-5-2
7-6-1

Fig. 7-6-2 (400×)
Same patient as in fig. 7-6-1. L.C.S.F. Carcinoma recti.
A differentiation between carcinoma recti and carcinoma coli is impossible (see figs. 7-5-1/7-5-2).

Fig. 7-6-3 (400×)
Same patient as in fig. 7-6-2. L.C.S.F. Carcinoma recti.
Obvious polymorphism of nuclei.

Fig. 7-6-4 (400×)
Same patient as in fig. 7-6-1. L.C.S.F. Carcinoma recti.
Differential diagnosis with an arachnoidea tissue sheet may be difficult. There is, however, a signet ring cell and the cytoplasm is very light blue.

Fig. 7-7-1 (400×)
Patient B. L.C.S.F. Carcinoma of the pancreas. The tumor diagnosis is evident because of the anisokaryosis and anisocytosis. The cytoplasm is light-blue and granulated.

7-6-2

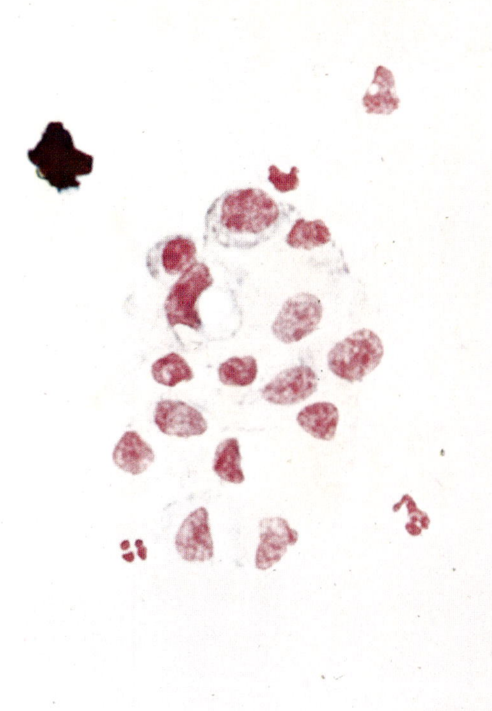

7-6-3

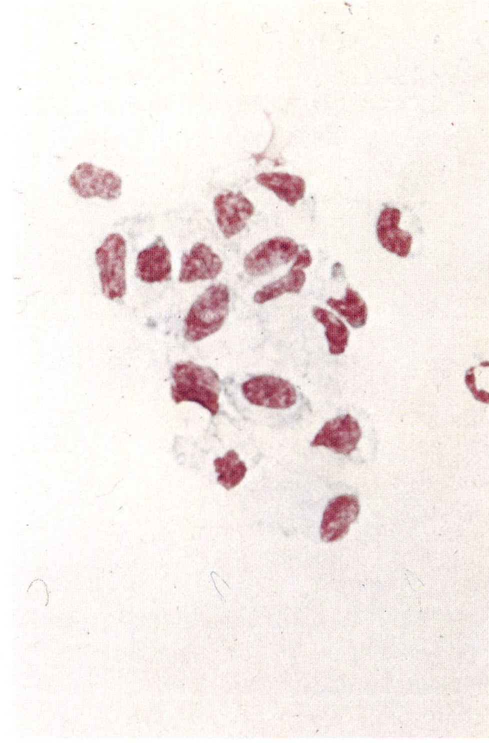

7-6-4

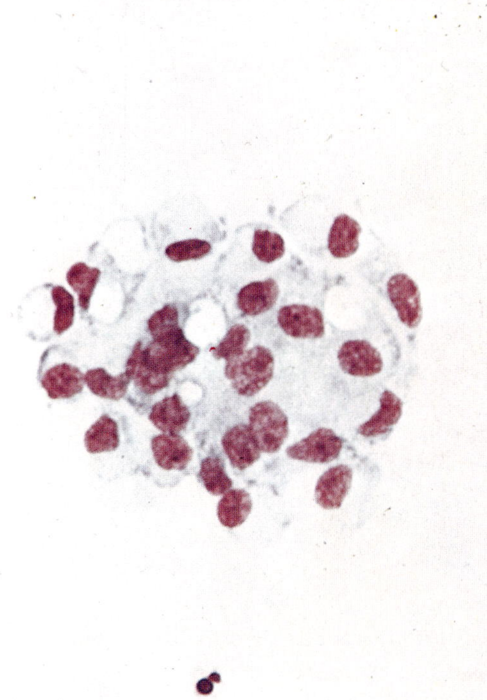

7-7-1

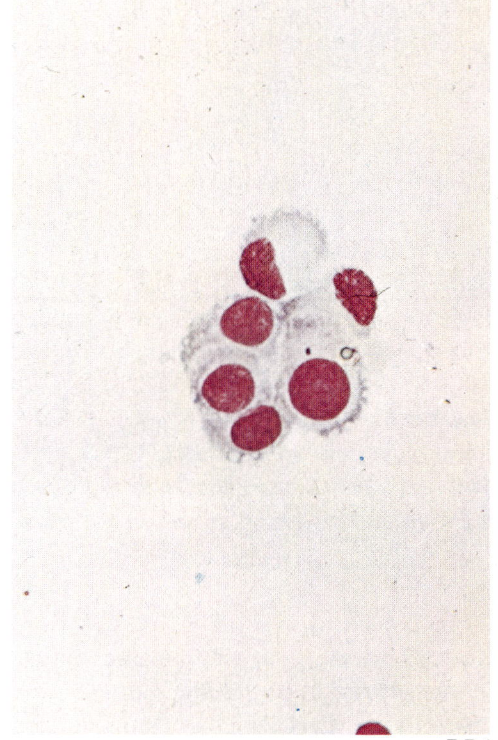

Fig. 7-7-2 (400×)
Same patient as in fig. 7-7-1. L.C.S.F. Carcinoma of the pancreas. Tumor sheet
with 2 cells. One is a typical signet ring cell while the other has vacuoles.

Fig. 7-7-3 (400×)
Same patient as in fig. 7-7-1. L.C.S.F. Carcinoma of the pancreas. A tumor
diagnosis on these cells is impossible although they are from the same spinal
fluid specimen of figs. 7-7-1 and 7-7-2 and the cells are of the same type.

Fig. 7-8-1 (400×)
Patient v.R. L.C.S.F. Melanoma. The left eye was the primary site.
One melanoma cell and one lymphocyte. In the cytoplasm are very fine grey
melanin granules. There are two nuclei of unequal size.

Fig. 7-8-2 (625×)
Same patient as in fig. 7-8-1. L.C.S.F. Melanoma. Three free lying melanoma
tumor cells with anisokaryosis and melanin granules.

Fig. 7-8-3 (625×)
Same patient as in fig. 7-8-1. L.C.S.F. Melanoma.
Small tissue fragment with typical melanoma aspect.

Fig. 7-8-4 (625×)
Same patient as in fig. 7-8-1. L.C.S.F. Melanoma. Three different melanoma cells.
One of them is dark colored by melanin granules. The cells contain different
quantities of melanin granules.

Fig. 7-8-5 (625×)
Same patient as in fig. 7-8-1. L.C.S.F. Melanoma.
Three different melanoma cells. Same characteristics as in fig. 7-8-4. There is a
marked anisocytosis and anisokaryosis.

Fig. 7-8-6 (625×)
Same patient as in fig. 7-8-1. L.C.S.F. Melanoma.
A macrophage filled with melanin. Because of the normal inactive nucleus this is
not a tumor cell. In the macrophages the melanin granules are always more
coarse in contrast with the finer granules in the tumor cells.

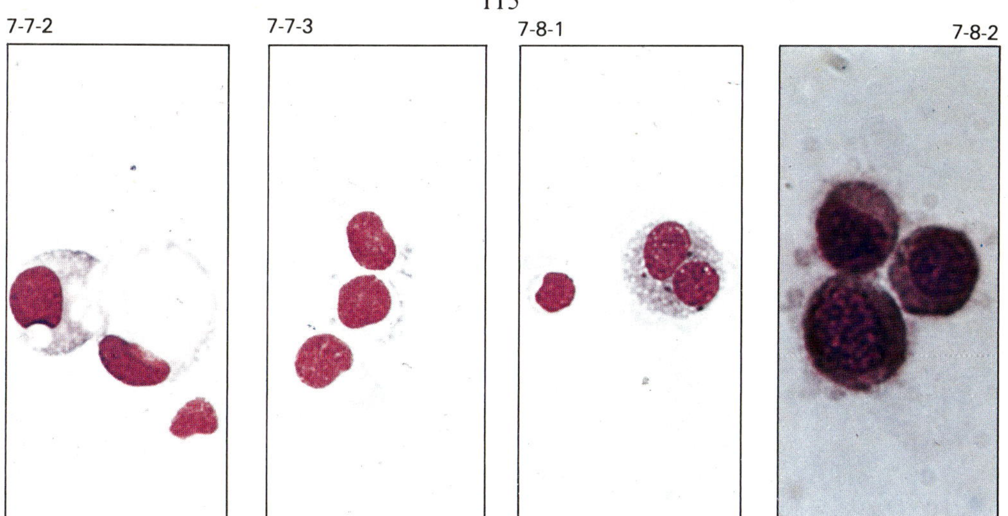
7-7-2
7-7-3
7-8-1
7-8-2

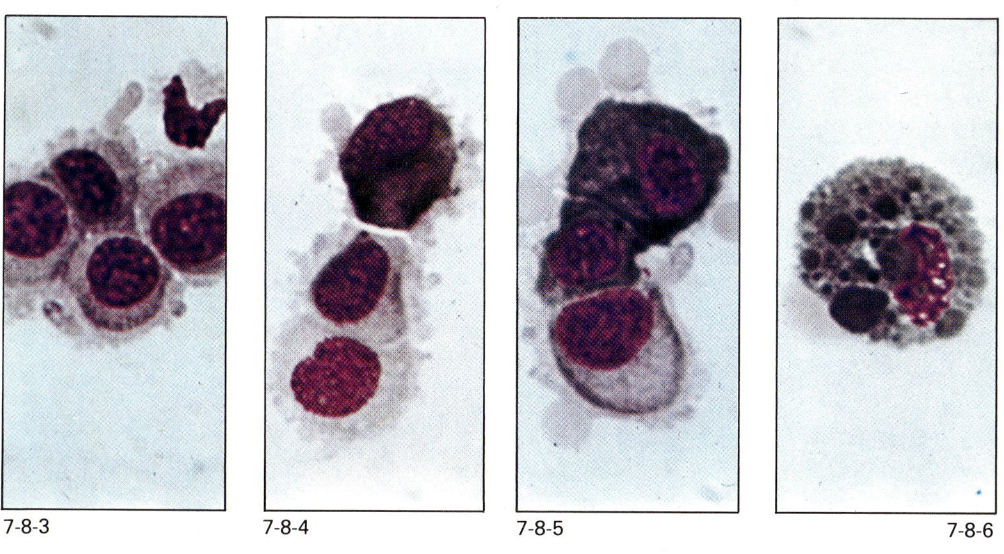
7-8-3
7-8-4
7-8-5
7-8-6

Fig. 7-8-7 (625 ×)
Patient Sj. L.C.S.F. Melanoma. Tissue sheet of tumor cells. P.A. diagnosis
melanoma. There are only a few dark melanin granules.

Fig. 7-8-8 (625 ×)
Patient Ray. L.C.S.F. Melanoma. Giant tumor cells of a malignant melanoma
without melanin (leuco-form).

Fig. 7-9-1 (625 ×)
Patient G. L.C.S.F. Retinoblastoma. Tissue sheet of tumor cells showing very
large nuclei and prominent nucleoli. There is dense crowding of the nuclei. The
nucleus-cytoplasm ratio is very high. There are multiple mitoses.

Fig. 7-9-2 (625 ×)
Same patient as in fig. 7-9-1. L.C.S.F. Retinoblastoma. There is less crowding
and a more regular tissue structure. This tissue fragment resembles a
medulloblastoma.

Fig. 7-9-3 (625 ×)
Same patient as fig. 7-9-1. L.C.S.F. Retinoblastoma. Marked polymorphism of the
nuclei. Cells grouped in the form of a palisade.

7-8-7

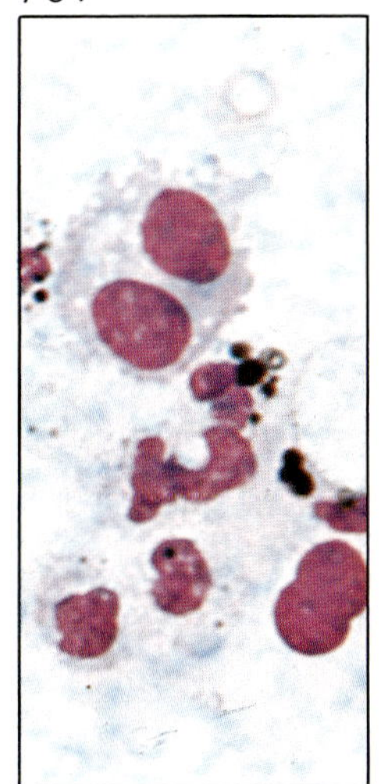

7-8-8

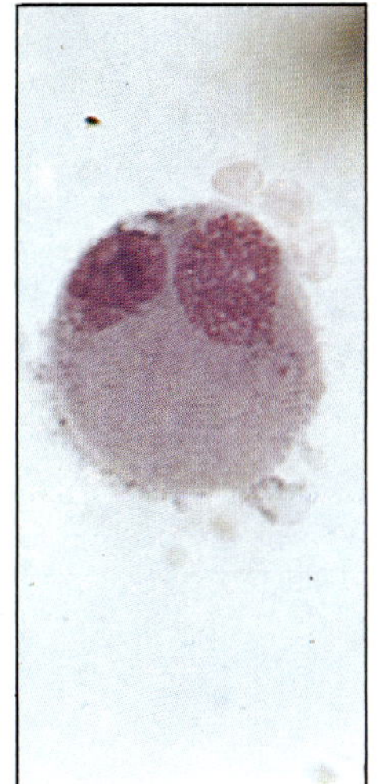

7-9-1

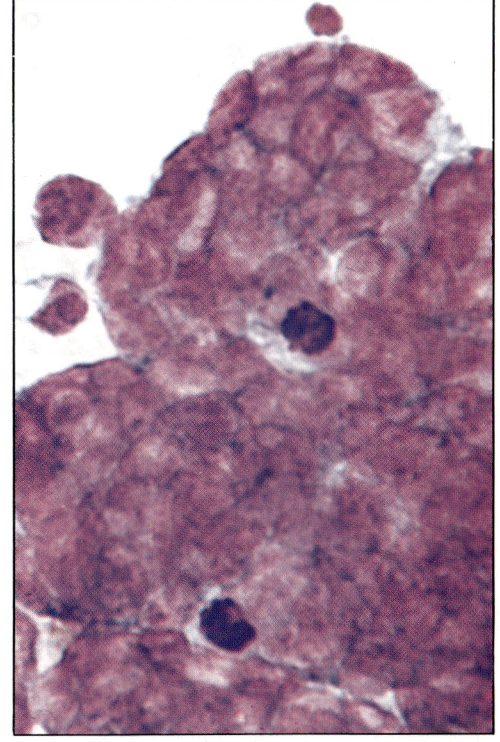

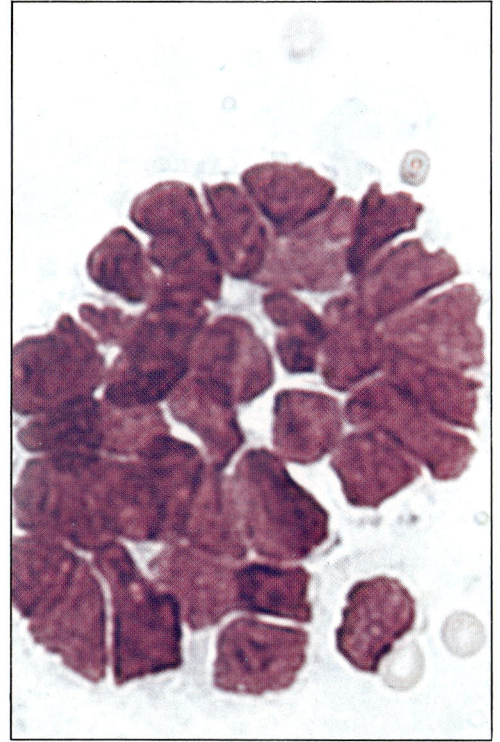

7-9-2

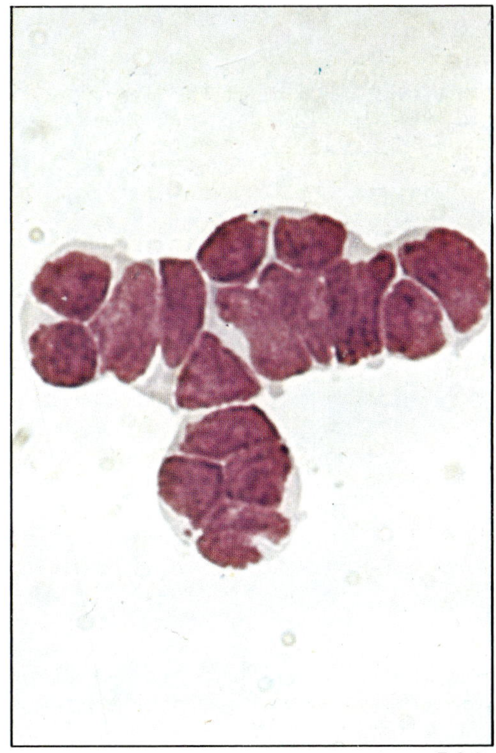

7-9-3

Fig. 7-9-4 (625 ×)
Same patient as fig. 7-9-1. L.C.S.F. Retinoblastoma. Bizarre nuclear morphology.
Rosette formation.

Fig. 7-10-1 (625 ×)
Patient H. L.C.S.F. Neuroblastoma. Tumor of conus and cauda equina.
Three cells with anisokaryosis.

Fig. 7-10-2 (625 ×)
Same patient as in fig. 7-10-1. L.C.S.F. Neuroblastoma. Tumor of conus and
cauda equina. Tissue sheet with dark relatively uniform nuclei. The cytoplasm is
violet-blue.

Fig. 7-10-3 (625 ×)
Same patient as in fig. 7-10-1. L.C.S.F. Neuroblastoma.
Tumor of conus and cauda equina. An other tissue sheet with slight
anisokaryosis. Nuclear membrane irregularities and hyperchromasia.

Fig. 7-10-4 (625 ×)
Same patient as in fig. 7-10-1. L.C.S.F. Neuroblastoma.
Tumor of conus and cauda equina. A tissue sheet with rosette formation.
The cytology is almost identical with the P.A.preparation.

7-9-4

7-10-1

7-10-2

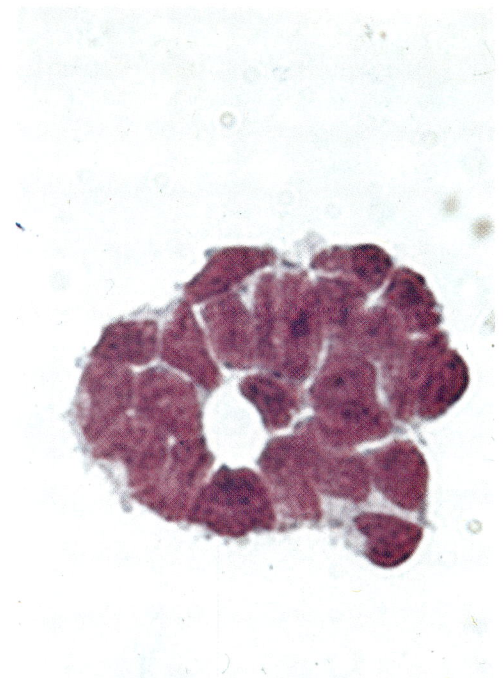

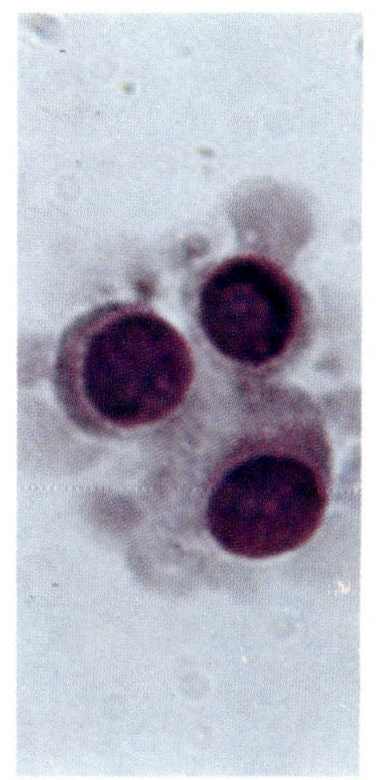

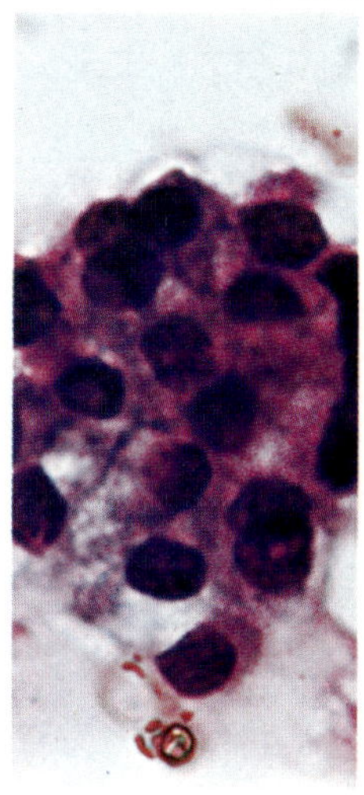

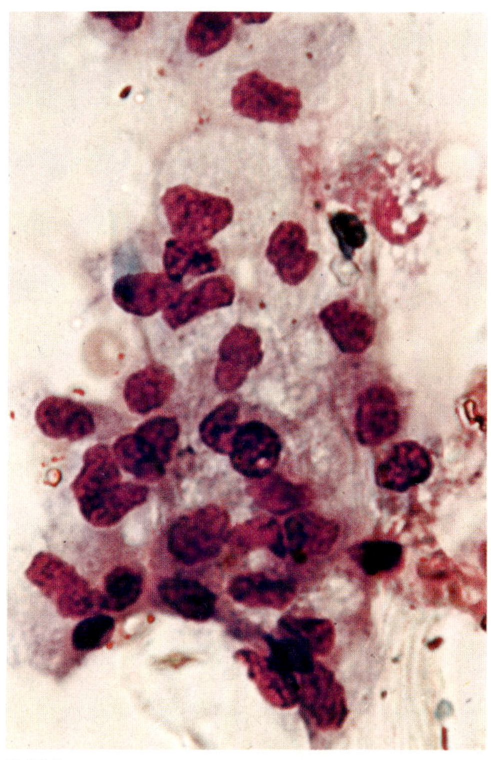

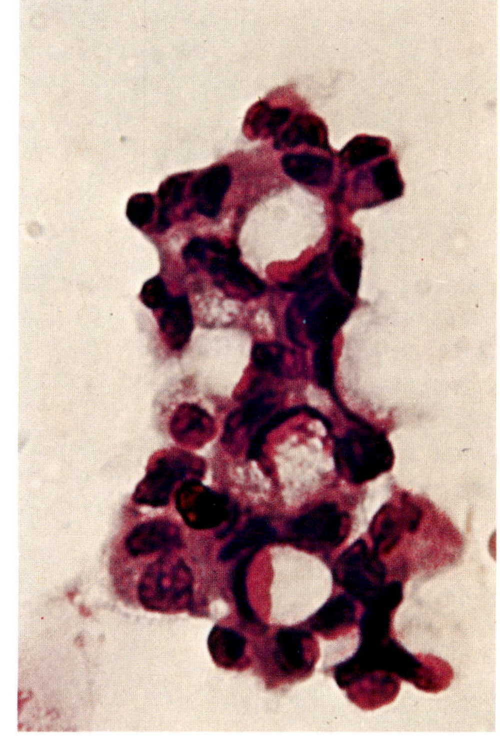

7-10-3

7-10-4

Fig. 8-1-1 (625×)
Patient de J. L.C.S.F. Reticulosarcoma. Typical characteristics of malignancy.
Anisocytosis and anisokaryosis. The cytoplasm has the same color as a
squamous cell carcinoma.

Fig. 8-1-2 (625×)
Same patient as in fig. 8-1-1. L.C.S.F. Reticulosarcoma. Same picture as fig. 8-1-1.
Nuclear membrane irregularities.

Fig. 8-1-3 (625×)
Same patient as in fig. 8-1-1. L.C.S.F. Reticulosarcoma. Bizarre nuclei.

Fig. 8-1-4 (625×)
Same patient as in fig. 8-1-1. L.C.S.F. Reticulosarcoma. Prominent nucleoli.
Hyperchromasia. A specific diagnosis on this preparation is impossible.

8-1-1

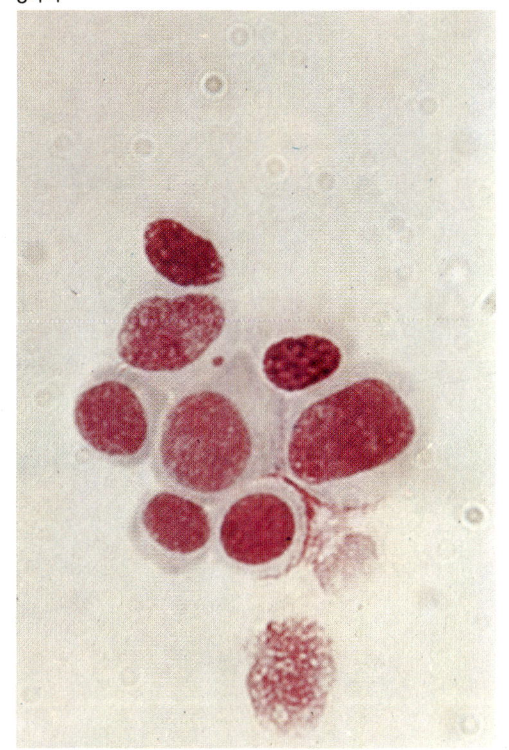

8-1-2

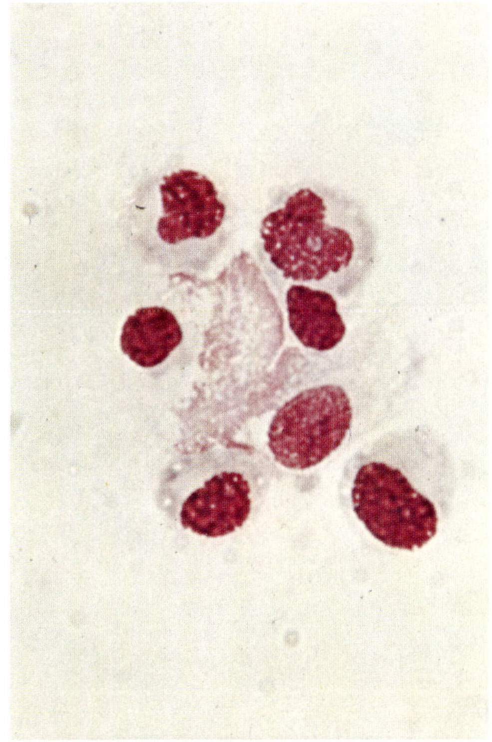

8-1-3

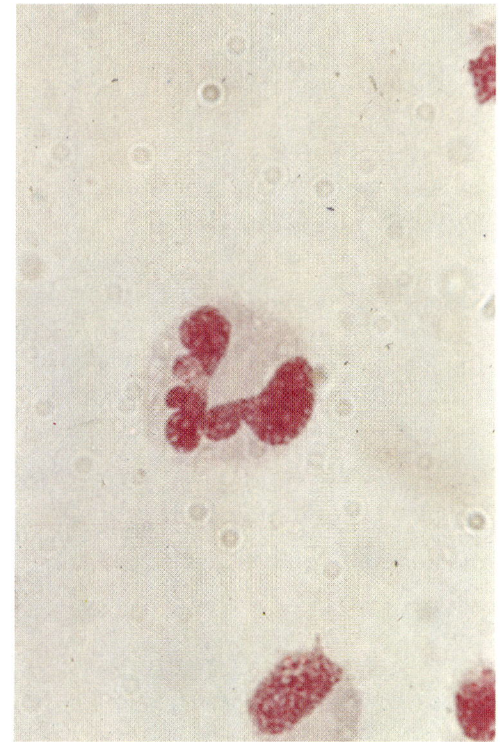

8-1-4

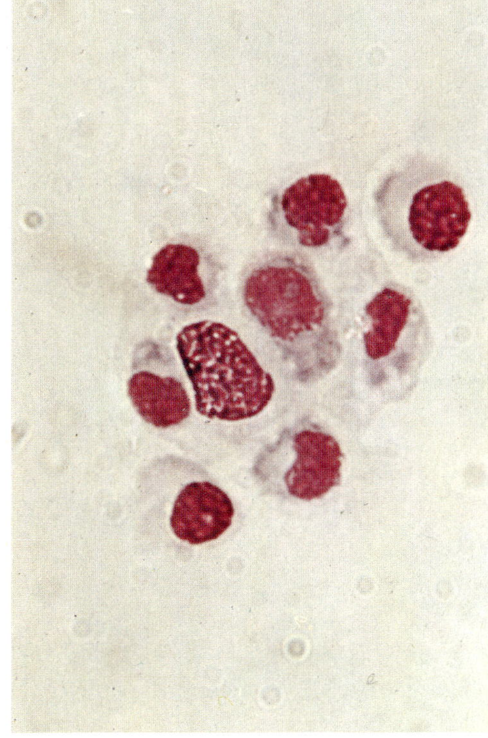

Fig. 8-1-5 (625 ×)
Patient v.d.M. L.C.S.F. Non-Hodgkin lymphoma. (T lymphocytic lymphoma).
Crowding of nuclei. Picture as in medulloblastoma or retinoblastoma.
One cell in mitosis.

Fig. 8-1-6 (625 ×)
Same patient as in fig. 8-1-5. Non Hodgkin lymphoma. (T lymphocytic lymphoma).
Completely different morphology. Dark blue-violet cytoplasm. Two giant tumor
cells with polymorphism of nuclei. Multiple nuclei and hyperchromasia.

Fig. 8-1-7 (1000 ×)
Patient B. L.C.S.F. Non Hodgkin lymphoma. Many isolated cells. The cytoplasm
is light-blue. The nuclei show pronounced differences in size and shape, and are
bizarre. Resemblance with leukemic cells.

Fig. 8-1-8 (1000 ×)
Patient B. L.C.S.F. Non Hodgkin lymphoma. Free lying cells. The shape of the
nuclei is bizarre.

8-1-5

8-1-6

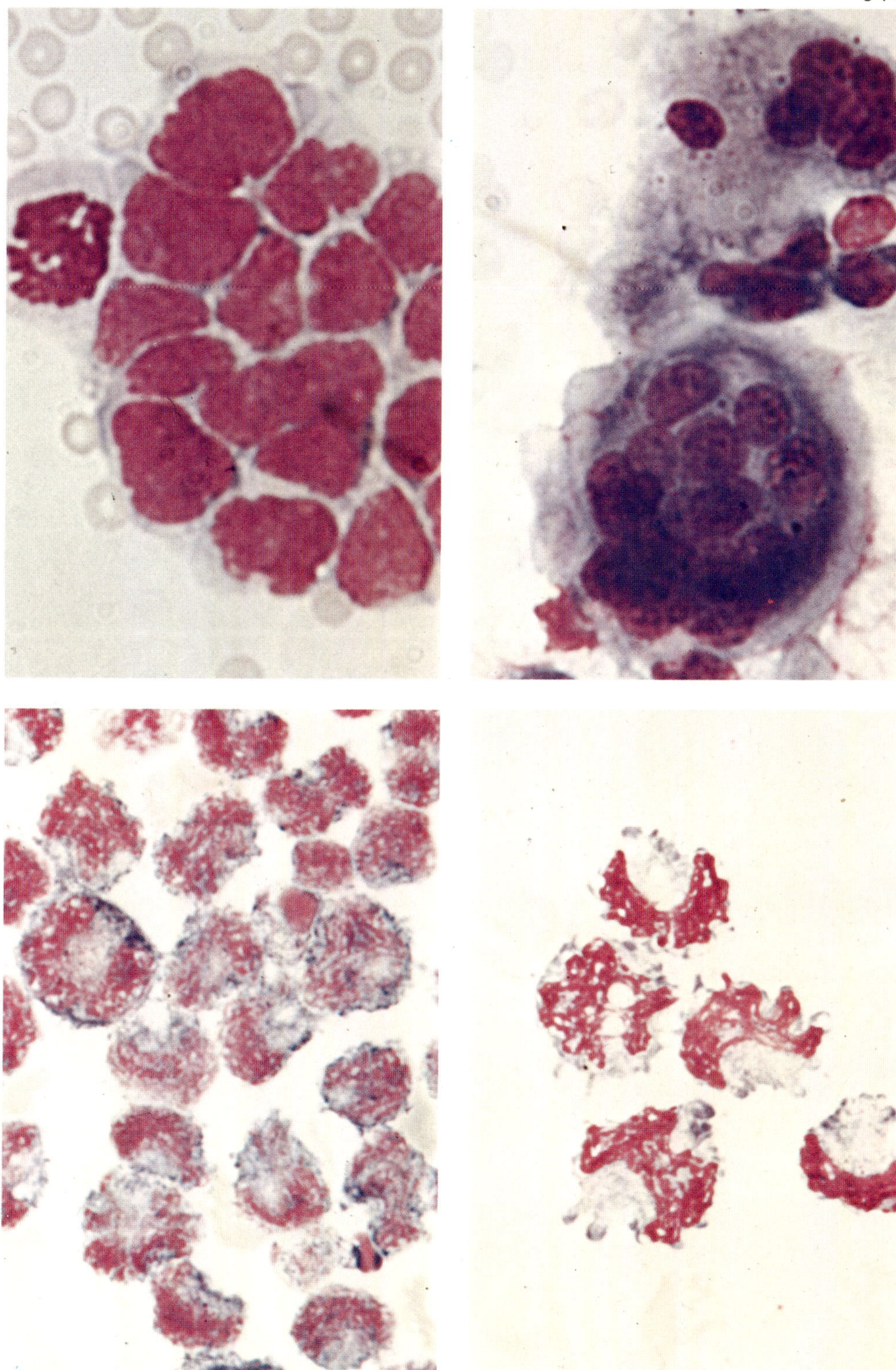

8-1-7

8-1-8

Fig. 8-1-9 (1000 ×)
Patient B. L.C.S.F. Non Hodgkin lymphoma. α-naphtylacetate esterase staining
is positive. The cells are, therefore, monoblasts. This is contrary to findings in
fig. 8-1-10. (Courtesy R. Goudsmit, M.D.)

Fig. 8-1-10 (1000 ×)
Patient B. L.C.S.F. Non Hodgkin lymphoma. Sudan Black-PAS staining.
The cells are Sudan black positive (brown granulation) and PAS positive.
Differentiation between lymphoblasts and myeloblasts is impossible. (Courtesy
R. Goudsmit, M.D.)

Fig. 8-2-1 (625 ×)
Patient D. Chronic lymphatic leukemia. L.C.S.F.
The white blood cells are larger than normal and present in an enormous
amount.
The nucleus-cytoplasm ratio has changed in favor of the nuclei.
The nuclei are carved and relatively uniform.

Fig. 8-2-2 (625 ×)
Same patient as fig. 8-2-1. Chronic lymphatic leukemia. L.C.S.F.
There is slightly more polymorphism and a mitosis.

8-1-9
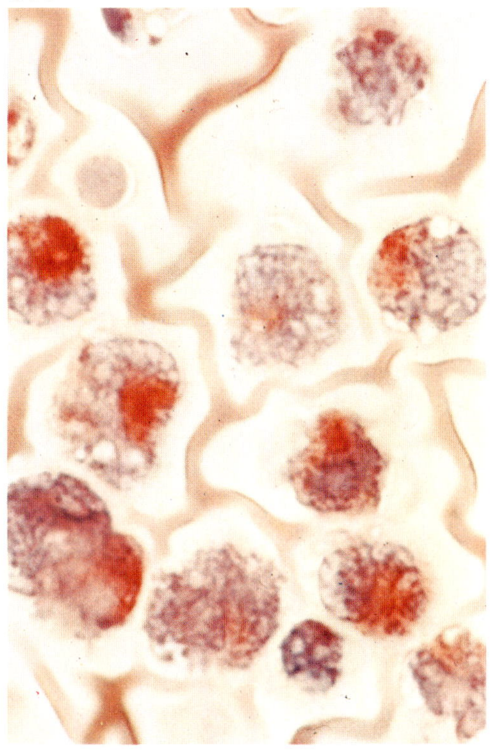

8-1-10
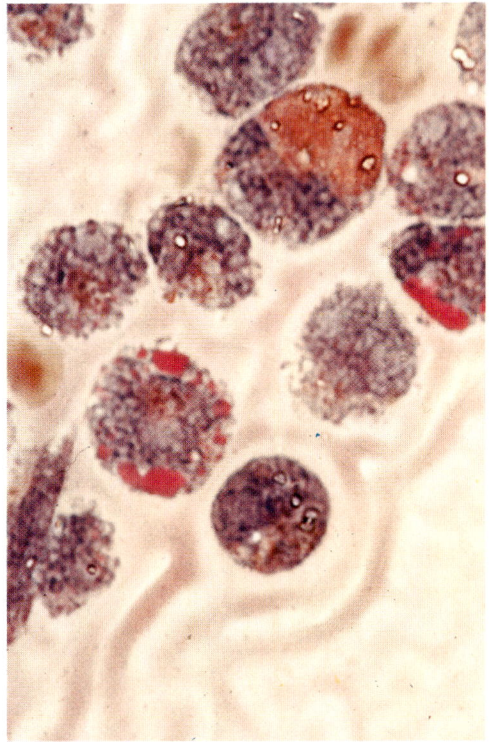

8-2-1
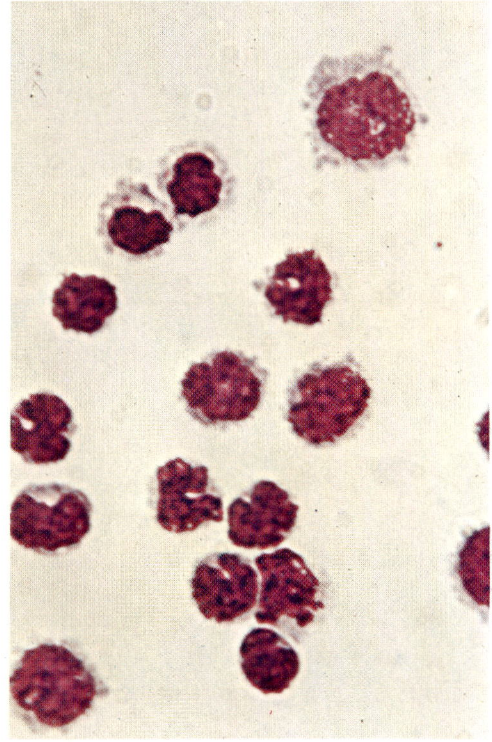

8-2-2
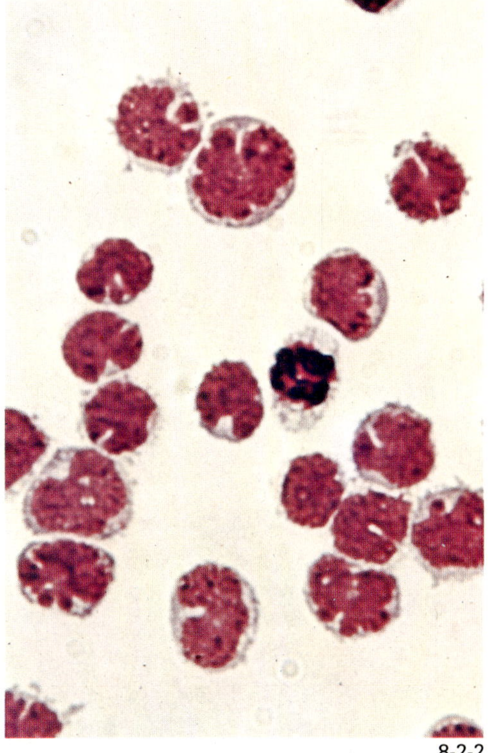

Fig. 8-3-1 (625×)
Patient B. Acute myeloid leukemia. L.C.S.F. There is more polymorphism than in chronic lymphatic leukemia.

Fig. 8-3-2 (625×)
Same patient as in fig. 8-3-1. Acute myeloid leukemia. L.C.S.F.
There is a pronounced anisokaryosis and anisocytosis.

Fig. 10-1-1 Case for diagnosis.
Patient G. V.C.S.F. Hydrocephalus. Monro occlusion. Etiology unknown.
Macrophage phagocytosing plasma cells.

Fig. 10-1-2 Case for diagnosis.
Patient v.d.S. L.C.S.F. Meningitis carcinomatosa.
Primary site unknown.

8-3-1

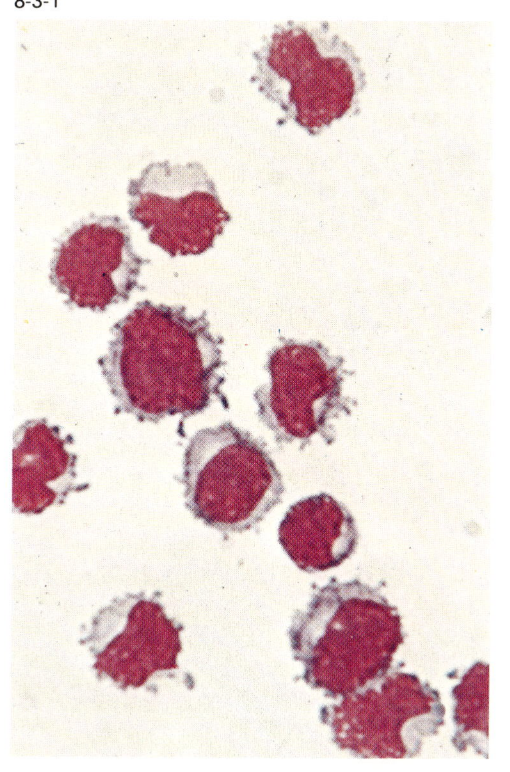

8-3-2

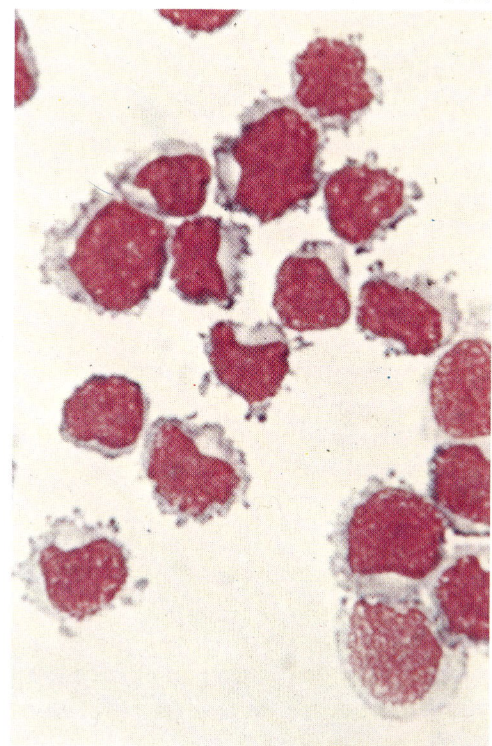

10-1-1

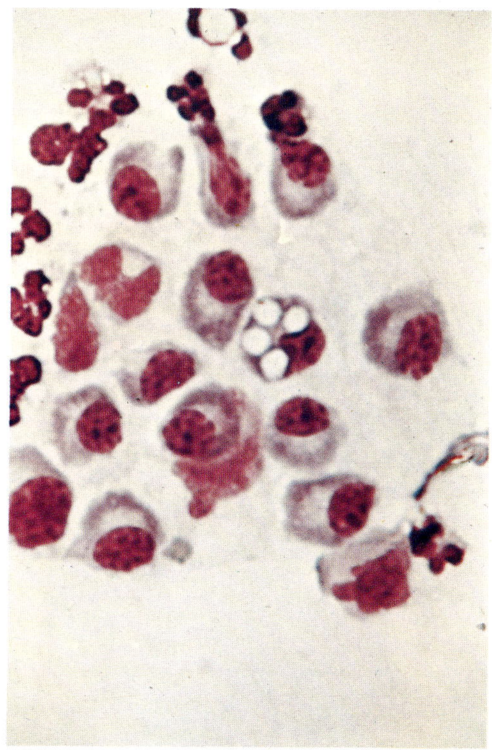

10-1-2

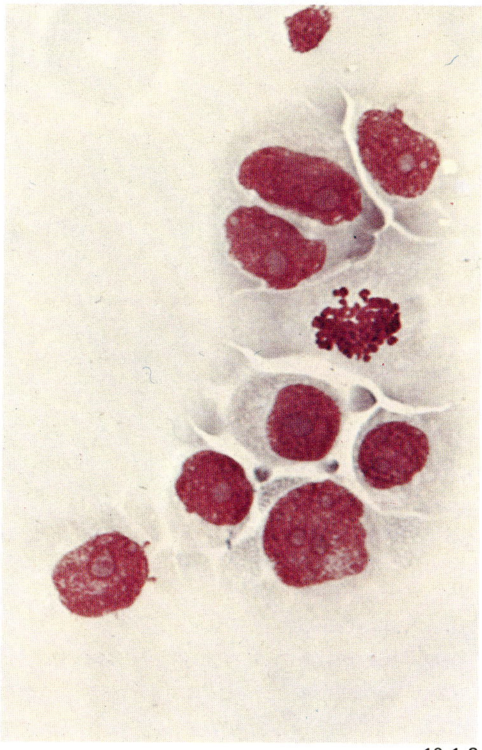

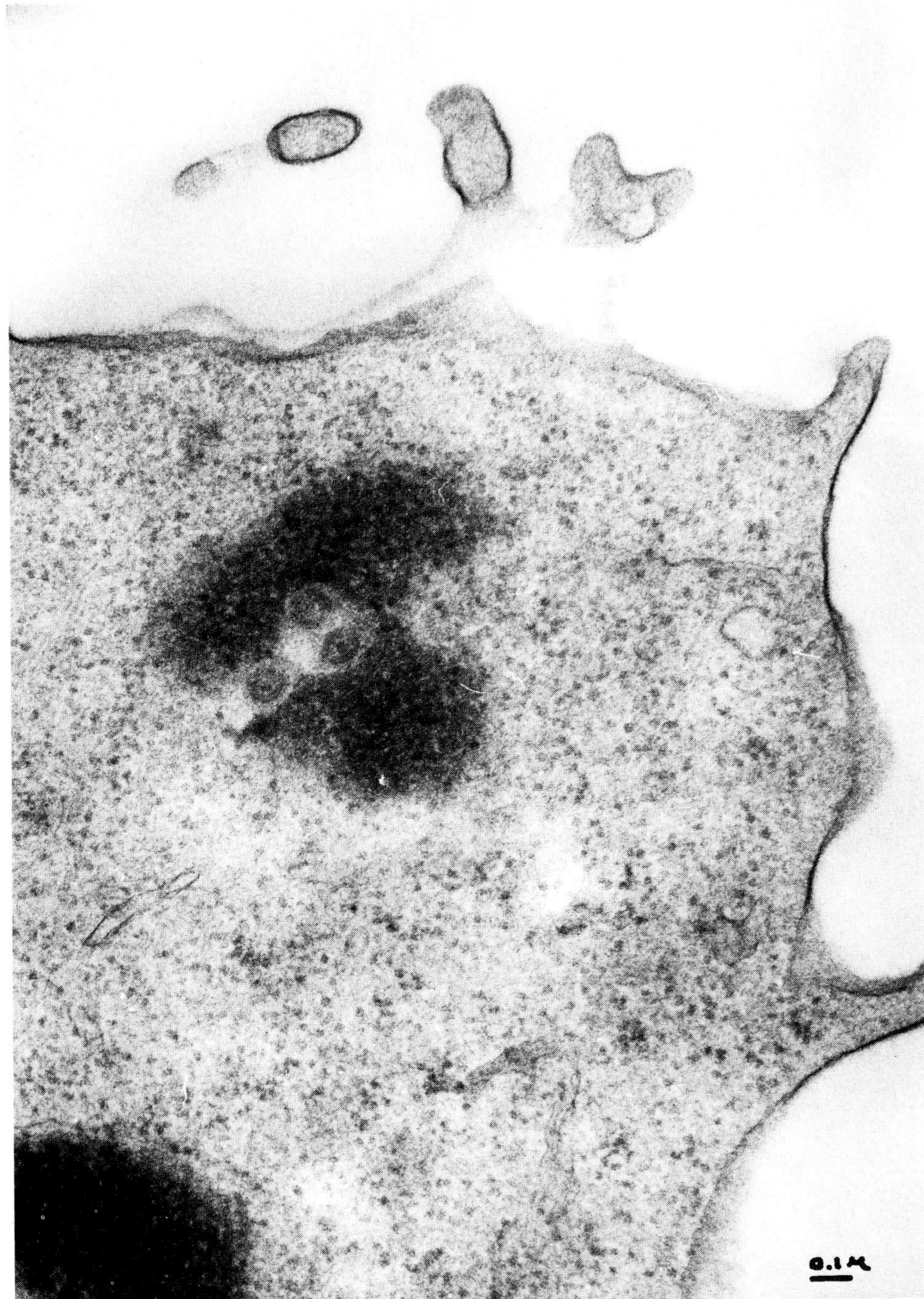

Plate 1-1
Electron micrograph 64.400 ×.
Clinical diagnosis: meningo-encephalitis in mononucleosis infectiosa.
Herpes-like particles with a central core in a C.S.F. cell (Epstein-Barr virus).
Unpublished observation from the author.

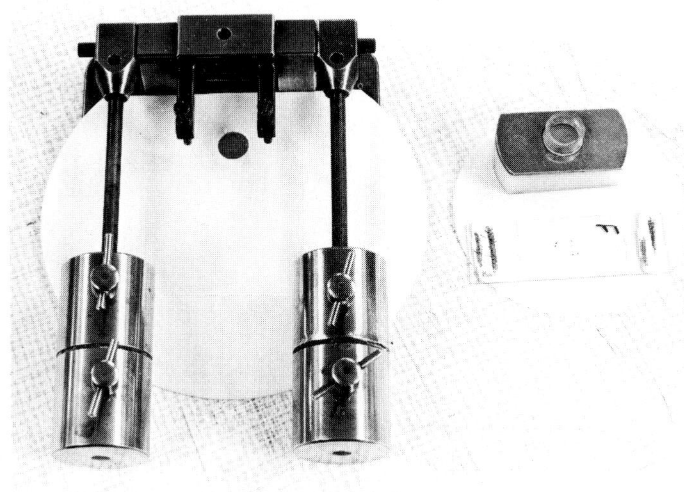

Plate 9-1
A Sayk model sedimentation chamber.
Front view.

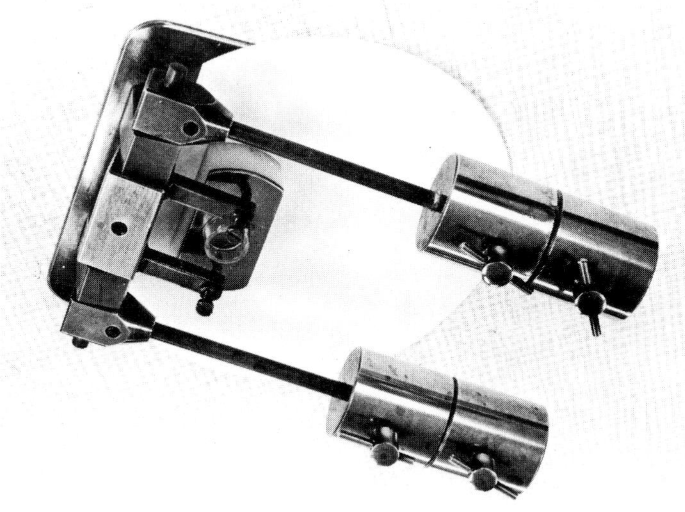

Plate 9-2
A Sayk model sedimentation chamber ready for use.
Side view.

References

Baringer, J.R.
A simplified procedure for spinal fluid cytology. Arch.Neurol.(Chic.) **22**: 305–308 (1970).

Bischoff, A.
Erfahrungen mit der Tumorzelldiagnostik im Liquor cerebrospinalis. Acta neurochir.(Wien) **9**: 510–524 (1961).

Bots, G.T.A.M., Went, L.N. and Schaberg, A.
The results of a sedimentation technique for cytology of cerebrospinal fluid. Acta cytol.(Philad.) **8**: 234–241 (1964).

Boyd, J.F. and Vince-Ribaric, V.
The examination of cerebrospinal fluid cells by fluorescent antibody staining to detect mumps antigen. Scand.J.infect.Dis. **5**: 7–15 (1973).

Brucher, J.M., Smidts, M. and J. Lecuit.
L'analyse cytologique du liquide céphalo-rachidien par une méthode de cytocentrifugation. Acta neurol. belg. **72**: 201–214 (1972).

Dayan, A.D. and Stokes, M.I.
Immunofluorescent detection of measles virus antigens in cerebrospinal fluid cells in subacute sclerosing panencephalitis. Lancet **I**: 891–892 (1971).

Dayan, A.D. and Stokes, M.I.
Rapid diagnosis of encephalitis by immunofluorescent examination of cerebrospinal fluid cells. Lancet **I**: 405–406 (1972)

Den Hartog Jager, W.A.
Cytopathology of the cerebrospinal fluid examined with the sedimentation technique after Sayk. J.neurol.Sci. **9**: 155–177 (1969).

De Vries, S.I. and Schreuder-van Gelder, R.
De betekenis van cytochemische kleuringen voor de diagnostiek van leukemie. Ned.T.Geneesk. **116**: 1008–1013 (1972).

Duffy, P.E., Simon, J., Defendini, R. and Karalion, S.
The study of cells in C.S.F. by electron microscopy. A new method. Arch. Neurol. (Chic.) **21**: 358–362. (1969).

Dufresne, J.J.
Praktische Zytologie des Liquors. Documenta Geigy, Basel (1973).

Gardner, P.S. and MacQuillin, J.
Rapid Virus Diagnosis. Application of Immunofluorescence. Butterworths, London (1974).

Greger, J. and Wieczorek, V.
Über das Vorkommen von Plasmazellen im Liquor cerebrospinalis bei neurologischen Erkrankungen.
Wien.Z.Nervenh. 23: 366–374 (1966).

Herndon, R.M. and Johnson, M.J.
A method for the electron microscopic study of cerebrospinal fluid sediment. J.Neuropath.exp.Neurol.
29: 320–330 (1970).

Herndon, R.M., Johnson, R.T., Davis, L.E. and Descalzi, L.R.
Ependymitis in mumps virus meningitis. Electron microscopical studies of C.S.F. Arch.Neurol.(Chic.)
30: 475–479 (1974).

Jarrat, M. and Hubler, W.R.
Herpes genitalis and aseptic meningitis. Arch.Derm. 110: 771–772 (1974).

Kaplow, L.S. and Burstone, M.S.
Cytochemical demonstration of acid phosphatase in hematopoietic cells in health and in various
hematological disorders using azo dye techniques. J.Histochem.Cytochem. 12: 805–811 (1964).

Kistler, G.S.
Zur Membranfilter-Technik in der Cytodiagnostik des Liquor cerebrospinalis. Nervenarzt 41: 507–510
(1970).

Kistler, G.S. and Bischoff, A.
Zur exfoliativen Cytologie kleiner Flüssigkeitsmengen. Schweiz.med.Wschr. 92: 863–866 (1962).

Kölmel, H.W.
Atlas of Cerebrospinal Fluid Cells. Springer-Verlag, Berlin-New York (1977).

Lee, F.K., Nahmias, A.J. and Stagno, S.
Rapid diagnosis of cytomegalovirus infection in infants by electron microscopy. New Engl.J.Med. 299:
1266–1270 (1978).

Lindeman, J., Müller, W.K., Versteeg, J. et al.
Rapid diagnosis of meningoencephalitis, encephalitis. Neurology (Minneap.) 24: 143–148 (1974).

Lopes Cardozo, P.
Atlas of Clinical Cytology. Targa, 's-Hertogenbosch (1975).

Marshall, W.J.S.
Herpes simplex encephalitis treated with idoxuridine and external decompression. Lancet II: 579–580
(1967).

McCormick, W.F. and Coleman, S.A.
A membrane filter technique for cytology of spinal fluid. Amer.J.clin.Path. 38: 191–197 (1962).

McCormack, L.J., Hazard, J.B., Gardner, W.J. and Klotz, J.G.
Cerebrospinal fluid changes in secondary carcinoma of meninges. Am.J.clin.Path. 23: 470 (1953).

Metzel, E.
Eine einfache Methode zur Untersuchung der cellulären Bestandteile der Cerebrospinalflüssigkeit. Arch.Psychiat.Nervenkr. **204**: 222–228 (1963).

Naylor, B.
Cytologic study of intracranial fluids. Acta cytol.(Philad.) **5**: 198–202 (1961a).

Naylor, B.
An exfoliative cytologic study of intracranial fluids. Neurology (Minneap.) **11**: 560–570 (1961b).

Ochmichen, M.
Cerebrospinal Fluid Cytology. Georg Thieme, Stuttgart (1976).

Palmer, El., Martin, M.L. and Gary, G.W.Jr.
The ultrastructure of disrupted herpes virus nucleocapsids. Virology **65**: 260–265 (1975).

Pearse, A.G.E.
Histochemistry. Churchill Livingstone, Edinburgh and London, **II**, 1383 (1972).

Peters, A.C.B.
CSF cell immunofluorescence and cytology in viral neurological disease. Thesis (private publication), Leiden (1979).

Peters, A.C.B. and Versteeg, J.
Unpublished data.

Peters, A.C.B., Versteeg, J., Bots, G.T.A.M. et al.
Varicella and acute cerebellar ataxia. Arch.Neurol.(Chic.) **35**: 769–771 (1978a).

Peters, A.C.B., Versteeg, J., Lindeman, J. et al.
Viral meningoencephalitis and head injury. Acta neurol.scand. **57**: 77–87 (1978b).

Peters, A.C.B., Versteeg, J., Bots, G.T.A.M. et al.
Nervous system complications of herpes zoster: immunofluorescent demonstration of varicella-zoster antigen in CSF cells. J.Neurol.Neurosurg. Psychiat. **42**: 452–457 (1979a).

Peters, A.C.B., Vielvoye, G.J., Versteeg, J. et al.
ECHO 25 focal encephalitis and subacute hemichorea. Neurology (Minneap.) **29**: 676–681 (1979b).

Peters, A.C.B., Versteeg, J., Bots, G.T.A.M. et al.
Progressive multifocal leukoencephalopathy: immunofluorescent demonstration of SV40 antigen in CSF cells and favourable response to cytarabine treatment. Submitted for publication (1979c).

Reynaud, A.J. and King, E.B.
A new filter for diagnostic cytology. Acta cytol. (Philad.) **11**: 289–294 (1967).

Rich, J.R.
A membrane filter technique for cerebrospinal fluid cytology. J.Neurosurg. **36**: 661–666 (1972).

Robbins, S.L.
Pathologic Basis of Disease. Saunders, Philadelphia, London, Toronto (1974).

Rubinstein, L.J.
Tumors of the central nervous system. Armed Forces Institute of Pathology, Washington D.C. (1972).

Russell, D.A. and Rubinstein, L.J.
Pathology of Tumours of the Nervous System. Edward Arnold Publ., London. Third edition (1971).

Sayk, J.
Ergebnisse neuer liquorcytologische Untersuchungen mit dem Sedimentierkammerverfahren. Ärztl.Wsch. **9**: 1042 (1954).

Sayk, J.
Cytologie der Zerebrospinalflüssigkeit. Fischer, Jena (1960).

Sayk, J.
The cerebrospinal fluid in brain tumors. Handbook of Clinical Neurology. Ed.P.J.Vinken and G.W. Bruyn, Vol. 16, Tumours of the Brain and Skull, Part I. North-Holland Publ. Co., Amsterdam 360–417 (1974).

Shoji, H., Koya, M. and Ogiwara, H.
Meningitis associated with herpes zoster. J. Neurol. **213**: 269–271 (1976).

Sommerville, R.G.
Rapid identification of neurotropic viruses by an immunofluorescent technique applied to cerebrospinal cellular deposits. Arch.ges.Virusforsch. **19**: 63–69 (1966).

Spaar, F.W. and Munz, E.
Ein einfaches Verfahren zur raschen Gewinnung von Liquorcellen für die cytologische Untersuchung. Nervenarzt **41**: 36–40 (1970).

Spriggs, A.I.
Malignant cells in cerebrospinal fluid. J.clin.Path. **7**: 122–130 (1954).

Spriggs, A.I. and Boddington, M.M.
The Cytology of Effusion. (Pleural, Pericardial and Peritoneal and of C.S.F.). Heineman, London, Second edition (1968).

Stefanko, St. and Kaluza, J.
La cytologie du liquide céphalo-rachidien dans les tumeurs du système nerveux. Schw.Arch.Neurol. Neurochir.Psychiat. **110**: 249–259 (1972).

Stokes, H.B., O'Hara, C.M., Buchanan, R.D. and Ollson, W.H.
An improved method for examination of cerebrospinal fluid cells. Neurology (Minneap.) **25**: 901–906 (1975).

Taber, L.H., Mirkovic, R.R., Adam, V. et al.
Rapid diagnosis of enterovirus meningitis by immunofluorescent staining of CSF leukocytes. Intervirology **1**: 127–134 (1973).

Taber, L.H., Brasier, F., Couch, R.B. et al.
Diagnosis of herpes simplex virus infection by immunofluorescence. J. clin. Microbiol. **3**: 309–312 (1976).

Tutuarima, J.A., Hische, E.A.H. and Van Der Helm, H.J.
An improved method for the concentration of cerebrospinal fluid cells by suction tip and sedimentation chamber. J. neurol.Sci. **44**: 61–67 (1979).

Wesemann, W.
Methodischer Beitrag zur Liquorcytodiagnostik. Dtsch.Z.Nervenheilk. **191**: 360–366 (1967).

Widal, J., Sicard, L. and Ravaut, G.
Cytologie du liquide céphalo-rachidien au cours de quelques processus méninges chroniques. Bull.Soc.méd.Hôp.Paris, 3 sér. **18**: 31 (1901).

Wieczorek, V.
Erfahrungen mit der Tumorzelldiagnostik in Liquor cerebrospinalis bei primären und metastatischen Hirngeschwülsten. Dtsch.Z.Nervenheilk. **186**: 410 (1964).

Wieczorek, V. and Greger, J.
Erfahrungen mit der Liquorzellendiagnostik. Eine Analyse von etwa 5000 liquorzytologische Untersuchungen. Psychiat.et Neurol. (Basel) **150**: 42–155 and 105–117 (1965).

Wilkins, R.H. and Odom, G.L.
Cytological changes in cerebrospinal fluid associated with resections of intracranial neoplasm. J.Neurosurg. **25**: 24–36 (1966).

Index